A Physician's Guide to Coping with Death and Dying

A Physician's Guide to Coping with Death and Dying

Jan Swanson and
Alan Cooper

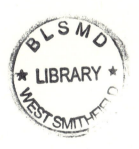

McGILL-QUEEN'S UNIVERSITY PRESS
Montreal & Kingston • London • Ithaca

© McGill-Queen's University Press 2005
ISBN 0-7735-2747-8 (cloth)
ISBN 0-7735-2832-6 (paper)

Legal deposit first quarter 2005
Bibliothèque nationale du Québec

Printed in Canada on acid-free paper that is 100% ancient forest free (100% post consumer recycled), processed chlorine free

McGill-Queen's University Press acknowledges the support of the Canada Council for the Arts for our publishing program. We also acknowledge the financial support of the Government of Canada through the Book Publishing Industry Development Program (BPIDP) for our publishing activities.

LIBRARY AND ARCHIVES CANADA CATALOGUING IN PUBLICATION

Swanson, Jan, 1948–
A physician's guide to coping with death and dying / Jan Swanson and Alan Cooper, 1947–
Includes bibliographical references and index.
ISBN 0-7735-2747-8 (bnd)
ISBN 0-7735-2832-6 (pbk)
1. Terminal care.   2. Physician and patient.   I. Cooper, Alan, 1947–   II. Title.
R726.8.S92 2005   616'.029   C813'.6   C2005-904449-4

Typeset in 10.5/13 Sabon with Syntax.
Book design and typesetting by zijn digital.

Contents

List of Figures and Tables

Preface

To everything, there is a season and a time to every purpose under heaven: a time to be born, and a time to die.

Ecclesiastes 3:1–8

A cardiologist told the residents on the ICU that he believed one of his patients, an even-tempered, kind man in his fifties, was dying: periodic bursts of severe pain dropped the patient's blood pressure dangerously low. The doctor, who had not told the patient he was dying, then left for the evening, leaving the residents, including Jan Swanson (referred to hereafter as JS), to care for his patient.

The residents knew the evening would be busy and that several patients in very critical condition might die. With almost no time for breaks, the residents dashed to the cafeteria for a quick meal. While eating, JS could think of nothing but the good man upstairs in a sterile hospital room, alone and close to death. Later, she wished she had skipped dinner and stayed with that man in his final moments. She still feels that the hospital failed someone who desperately needed the support of just one other human being on the night of his death.

Sometimes physicians talk around the subject of death, without really acknowledging it. Although they care, when they are faced with death, fear often prevents them from talking or makes them appear evasive.

The authors knew of an AIDS patient who was in an advanced stage of the disease. He had severe diarrhea, was badly dehydrated, and wasn't responding to aggressive treatment. Instead of telling the patient how critical the problem was and that death was a very real possibility, the attending physician dropped hints: "You shouldn't be getting transfusions. It's just a waste of money," and "It's probably best if you just go home."

The patient was hurt, as well he might have been. The physician, who was actually a caring man, appeared to be cold and unfeeling because he allowed his fear to take over when faced with any discussion about death.

When it comes to medical knowledge and technique, most physicians have it down. Take the subject of death out of the clinical realm, however, and most physicians are out in the cold. While they know what they should do, they don't know how to do it.

Most medical students and physicians receive no formal training dealing with death and the process of dying on a personal, emotional, or spiritual level. They have had no training that helps them talk about death with patients and their families. We believe that physicians and health professionals must address death directly, not ignore it, and have written A Physician's Guide to Coping with Death and Dying for the beginning health professional. We are aware that there is no single, correct answer to questions about treating a dying patient or the patient's family. We know, too, that there is no "best way" to tell patients when they have a potentially fatal illness.

The authors expect that medical students, residents, and physicians new to their practise will find this book helpful. More experienced physicians who were not trained to deal effectively with dying patients and their families or who want to learn ways to care for themselves while carrying out this difficult work may also find this book useful. Other health care professionals, including nurses, nurse practitioners, and physician-assistants who work with dying patients in their practices, may also seek some guidance. In short, this is an entry level guide that many experienced professionals will find interesting, if only to confirm and solidify what they already know.

Beliefs about death are intensely personal. Everyone, including health professionals, approaches death and dying with a distinct set of emotional, spiritual, and psychological frames of reference. The authors hope that this book will serve as a useful guide as health care professionals clarify their views and work with the widely divergent views of the patients, families, and physicians they encounter.

The authors have tried to paint a portrait that encompasses the wide range of cultural, emotional, spiritual, and psychological beliefs that dictate how people deal with the subjects of death and dying. The authors decided *not* to do an opinion poll. Instead they discussed the subject and questioned those with relevant knowledge who were willing to share their opinions.

The authors prepared questionnaires in four formats, asking those they questioned about their thoughts and beliefs about death and dying. The first format went to patients, a second to physicians, a third to families, and a fourth to friends of dying patients. Fifty-seven questionnaires were returned.

The patients and family members who answered the questionnaire knew the authors or had been referred to them by local health professionals. Most of these patients and their families had come in contact with death or with life-threatening illnesses. The physicians questioned were specialists in AIDS care or colleagues whom the authors knew. The authors chose ministers whose names appeared in the Dallas Yellow Pages church directory or who were associated with the National Interfaith Network, which had participated in a recent international conference on AIDS. All these people were quite honest in their responses. Since that time, seven of the respondents, including a physician, have died. The questionnaires provided a diversity of beliefs that can help physicians clarify their own responses.

This small study, which is not a scientific opinion poll, was meant to be exploratory, as the sample was not randomly selected and the questionnaire's psychometric properties were not investigated. The authors' intention was to generate a variety of opinions from some relevant people in the part of the US where the authors work.

While readers may not agree with all the beliefs and opinions presented, the authors hope that all readers will gain greater clarity about their own views.

It's not that I'm afraid to die. I just don't want to be there when it happens.
Woody Allen, *Getting Even*, 1971

PART ONE

Death and Dying

1

Understanding Death

Any man's death diminishes me, because I am involved in mankind; and therefore never send to know for whom the bell tolls; it tolls for thee.
John Donne (1572–1631), *Meditation XVII*

According to a Buddhist tale, a woman was unable to accept the death of her child. After asking many people in her village for help, she finally approached the Buddha, who said he could help her. Before he did so, though, she must bring him a mustard seed from a house in the village in which no one had ever died. She went from house to house, asking for the mustard seed, but could not find a single home untouched by death. When she finally returned to Buddha, she was empty handed. She knew the time had come to bury her child.

The subjects of death and dying are very recent additions to medical school curriculums. In 1980, 104 of 114 medical schools included a short session about death and dying, but nothing more extensive (Listen, 1975, Black et al., 1989, Hill, 1995, Johnson, 1996).

Death and dying still continue to receive little attention in the medical literature. In one controlled trial designed to improve care for seriously ill patients, nearly 60 per cent of the patients reported that they had no discussion with their physician regarding their prognosis or wishes for resuscitation (SUPPORT, 1995).

In a statement developed for the US National Consensus Conference on Medical Education for Care Near the End of Life, Susan Block and her colleagues from prestigious medical centres across the US (Block et al., 1998) expressed concern that "caring for dying patients is troublesome for many physicians. Physicians in general, including primary care physicians, feel inadequately prepared to care for the dying" (769). (McWhinney and Stewart, 1994, Von Gunten et al., 1994, Steinmetz et al., 1993, Schneiderman, 1997). Block and her colleagues proposed that primary care education and the entire range of medical education include and integrate the attitudes and skills necessary for high quality palliative care.

Because of the discomfort that many physicians feel, certain apparently irrelevant demographic characteristics predict whether physicians will withhold or withdraw life support when treating critically ill patients. These characteristics, which are associated with individual physicians and include their age, religion, the geographic location of their hospital and its type, appear to influence end-of-life care decisions. The characteristics, which do not reflect what the patient and family may want, are non-rational biases. They have no place in professional decision-making (Gilligan and Raffin, 1996, Raffin, 1995).

When asked to predict what patients would want for end-of-life care, physicians have little predictive power according to studies. Spouses and other intimates are also poor predictors (Seckler et al., 1991, Sulmasy et al., 1994). What is telling about physicians' predictions is that their predictions correlate more closely with what they would want than with what their patients want (Schneiderman et al., 1993).

Why do physicians find it difficult to talk about death? The existing end-of-life care literature suggests the following reasons. Physicians may:

- Be reminded of their own mortality when a patient dies
- Receive little guidance, because North American society rejects death and has developed no cultural guidelines to deal with the subject or talk about it openly.
- Lack knowledge about advance directives, training, and experience in delivering bad news. They also lack role models in end-of-life care.
- Fear being blamed for the death of a patient. Because of guilt or shame, they may avoid the patient's family or friends.
- Be unable to deal with the emotional responses of patients and family members.
- Fear not knowing all the answers.

- Not believe the child who is dying can handle that information. (Also, some parents forbid physicians to talk to the children about death.)
- Fear that they will destroy a patient's hope, if they tell the patient the truth, because the patients may believe the doctor has given up on them.
- Fear that if they tell already anxious patients that they are about to die, they will upset or depress them further.
- Be constrained when patients are elderly, because the adult children may have asked the doctors not to mention the imminent death
- Be aware of medical legal concerns.
- Have time constraints and economic disincentives.
- Be uncomfortable acknowledging impending death or to admit defeat by the enemy that is death, because they have been taught to focus on cure.
  (Steinmetz et al., 1992, Tinseley et al., 1994, Scheel and Lynn, 1988, McCue, 1995, Edlich and Kübler-Ross 1992, Morrison, 1998, Larson and Tobin, 2000, Quill, 2000, Siegler and Levin, 2000, Fallowfield, 2002, Rousseau, 2001, Covinsky et al., 2000, Wenrich et al., 2001).

Honest listening is one of the best medicines we can offer the dying and bereaved.

Jean Cameron, *Time to Live, Time to Die*, 1991

MEDICAL SCHOOLS OFFER LITTLE TRAINING ON HOW TO RESPOND EMOTIONALLY TO DEATH AND DYING

In 1997–1998, only 4 of 126 medical schools in the US required a course on caring for dying patients, according to the Project to Educate Physicians on End-of-Life Care (Emanuel, von Gunten, and Ferris, 1999). In addition, only 41 per cent of 7,657 residency programs polled offered instruction on end-of-life medical and legal issues (SUPPORT, 1995). It appears that education about death and dying has been put on the back burner or neglected completely. The American Society of Clinical Oncology (ASCO) established a task force on Barriers to Optimal End-of-Life Care by Oncologists, which concluded "There is a general consensus that many patients and physicians are reluctant to talk about death until dying is close at hand. Many physicians interpret disease progression and death as therapeutic failure ... physicians do not receive systematic education in the clinical and physiological aspects of caring for the terminally ill patient. Few courses emphasize this during the medical under-graduate years, and postdoctoral training programs are generally characterized by a 'learning on the job' approach" (*American Society of Clinical Oncology*, 1998, 1988, 1991).

According to the ASCO task force, doctors are not trained to man-age pain and symptoms, talk about an illness realistically and with-out destroying the patient's hope, or discuss death or other matters of similar importance with patients.

Most resident physicians and many physicians have limited expe-rience in making end-of-life care decisions, according to a task force report published by the *Journal of the American College of Cardiology* (King et al., 1998). This task force reported that only 5 out of 126 medical schools taught a separate course on caring for the dying. Another 1998 study by the Association of American Medical Colleges found that while 122 US medical schools included material on death and dying as one topic in a more general course, only 6 schools required end-of-life care as a separate course (Varner, 1998). An earlier study, which surveyed 7,048 residence programs on this subject, found that only 26 offered a course on end-of-life care (Hill, 1995).

These studies have helped national experts understand why many physicians lack the knowledge and skills to meet national guide-lines regarding good end-of-life care. Delese Wear (2002) comments poignantly, "If it is true that clinical faculty would never expect students to perform a procedure without first having them watch one, then practise it with close guidance, why would they assume that students can perform, [referring here to good end-of-life care] on their own and without support, one of the most difficult tasks physicians are asked to do?"

An expensive, multi-site study on the care of the dying in US hospitals actually embarrassed the American medical community. The Study to Understand Prognoses and Preferences for Outcomes and Risks of Treatment (SUPPORT) was conducted in two phases. Phase I, which examined data on 4,301 seriously ill patients, found physicians did not communicate well with their patients about treatment preference, including the aggressiveness of the treatment. For example, more than half of the doctors were unaware of their patients' do not resuscitate (DNR) preferences. Of the DNR orders in the patients' charts, almost half were written only within two days before the patients died (SUPPORT, 1995).

Phase II randomized 4,804 patients into intervention and control groups during a two-year period. For the intervention group, trained nurses were selected to initiate and provide physicians with early and accurate information about prognoses and families' preferences. No special efforts were made for the control group. No significant differences were found on the outcome variables, including how well physicians understood patients' preferences, the number of DNR orders, the number of days spent in an Intensive Care Unit (ICU), in a coma, or on a ventilator support machine, and the degree of pain reported (Oddi and Casey, 1998).

Although a majority of physicians favoured advance directives regarding end-of-life care in a previous study (Davidson et al., 1989), most physicians in the SUPPORT study remained unaware of their patients' wishes. For example, less than 50 per cent of physicians knew when their patients preferred that cardiopulmonary resuscitation be withheld. The American Medical Association responded to the SUPPORT study by proposing an end-of-life care program for physicians (Schneiderman, 1997, Emanuel et al., 1999).

Additional data from the SUPPORT study indicated that treatment of symptoms, such as pain, dyspnea, and profound weakness, require significant improvement. A medical record review of 9,105 seriously ill patients found that 55 per cent were conscious during the last three days of life; 40 per cent experienced severe pain; 80 per cent felt severe fatigue; and 63 per cent had difficulty with emotional or physical symptoms (King et al., 1998) Another study concerning training in end-of-life care (American Board of Internal Medicine, 1996) revealed that most directors of internal medicine residency programs found much lacking in this area of medical expertise. Also, a study's analysis of several medical textbooks revealed minimal information to help a physician (Carron et al., 1999).

"Death education" is a term applied to programs designed to improve the knowledge and understanding of the meaning of death, the process of dying, grief, and bereavement. These programs take one of two approaches. The cognitive/informative approach focuses on the acquisition of information, so the physician acquires some knowledge of the issues involved. The personal/affective approach attempts to help physicians understand their feelings about death, so they can deal more effectively and compassionately with the emotional, psychological, and spiritual issues experienced by their patients and their families. The latter approach helps physicians come to a better understanding of their own beliefs and values that pertain to death and the process of dying. The authors will use both approaches in this book (Kastenbaum and Kastenbaum, 1989).

WHY PHYSICIANS MUST UNDERSTAND AND FACE DEATH AND TALK TO THEIR PATIENTS ABOUT DEATH

Physicians must talk to patients about death and dying and allow them to express their fears openly. Too many patients are unable to discuss their fear of death because their physicians see no need to discuss the topic or are unable to do so.

Most physicians worry that if they discuss the withholding or withdrawing of care, their patients will become discouraged and give up on hope (Emanuel et al., 1991). In fact, the majority of patients involved in discussions of end-of-life directives are comforted by these conversations (La Puma and Moss, 1991). Another 1991 study reported that 80 per cent of patients wanted to discuss end-of-life care with their physicians; of those only 11 per cent reported engaging in such discussions. Patients initiated the majority of discussions (Gamble and Lichstein, 1991).

Physician and attorney Mark Garwin (1998) recommended that in a rapidly changing legal environment, a physician should initiate discussions about the risks involved in particular treatments and about the limits patients want placed on end-of-life care. He finds that most patients are reassured by these discussions and prefer their physician take the first step. He recommends that physicians initiate and document these discussions while the patients are still able to participate. He also suggests physicians follow their patients' wishes. By doing so, physicians will protect themselves legally when making future decisions (Garwin, 1998).

By speaking openly, physicians can help patients prepare for death and control the process (as much as medically possible). Patients can decide whom they want present at death and how loved ones can participate in the process.

In planning end-of-life care, physicians need to help their patients express their wishes early on, before they have lost the necessary clarity of mind. Although the spoken or written wishes of patients are valid, documents known as advance directives have gained popularity because their legal status is clearer. In these documents patients specify their wishes or name those who can make decisions for them. The advance directive is only needed, of course, when patients are unable to make end-of-life decisions. Patients retain the right to change their minds as often as they choose.

One limitation of advance directives, according to Garwin is that they are frequently nonspecific. Even the apparently specific term *do not resuscitate* can refer to many different interventions. Although often interpreted to forbid only cardiac massage, resuscitation could include electrical conversion of abnormal heart rhythms or administering oxygen, tracheal instruction, or drugs to correct problems with blood pressure or heart rhythm (Garwin, 1998).

JS treated the parents of a terminally ill leukemia patient who decided, after multiple treatments, to forego any more. Realizing he then had a very short time to live, he gathered together many of his friends and family who lived nearby and called those who lived out of state to inform them of his decision. After reviewing his will, he and his family decided to have a party. Not long after, he lapsed into a coma and died. His mother helped the hospice nurse bathe the body, thereby easing her sorrow. After the funeral, the mother and father told JS that the final get-together made their son's death less stressful. For the first time in years, members of the family felt at peace with one another.

When speaking of death, a good physician is able to discuss the risks and benefits associated with continuing treatment and the benefits to ending life. A 30-year-old man had terminal colon cancer, which had metastasized to his liver. His physicians provided him with data about the benefits and risks of treatment. He died at home with hospice care. By giving him this information, the physician helped him make an informed, meaningful, and appropriate decision.

In another case, a young woman had brain cancer. Her first surgeon told her the cancer was her fate; he did not recommend treatment. She decided to go to M.D. Anderson Cancer Center in Houston, Texas, at the advice of a physician friend. Even though her survival chances were slim, she decided to proceed with treatment. She sought a second opinion and tried an experimental treatment, making choices that fit her values and wishes. Nine years later, she is still alive.

Physicians who can deal with death and dying decrease their personal stress level and reduce the risk of burnout. One of the sadder moments JS witnessed as a medical student occurred when she witnessed her first birth. The baby, who had acute leukemia, began to die upon leaving his mother. Bleeding into all his organs, he screeched in pain. JS felt helpless, especially as she had never held a newborn infant before. The nurse told her to touch the child through the incubator. JS was grateful she could do something – anything. When the caring, understanding nurse told her what to do, the stress and guilt that JS felt decreased markedly.

Physicians who can deal with death and dying by using healthy coping mechanisms resist possible addiction. A physician, seemingly unaware of the inherent role conflict, cared for a close friend dying of AIDS. When the friend died, the physician turned to addictive drugs and began drinking heavily to cope with his loss. This doctor might have responded to loss in a less self-destructive way if he had recognized his boundaries and been more aware of his emotional limitations.

Physicians who can deal with death and dying are more compassionate and caring. By facing death, their own and that of others, physicians will more readily understand what patients and family members need. They will also be able to provide them with a sense of hope.

Physicians who are aware of their feelings about their own deaths and those of others are kinder to themselves and better able to heal themselves after losing patients. The authors once heard an AIDS expert talk about how sad and painful it was for him when AIDS patients, whom he had treated and to whom he had become very attached, died. Another doctor admitted to JS that when he dealt with AIDS patients, he felt as though he needed Prozac. These doctors were probably in touch with their feelings. They understood just how painful it could be to treat patients with terminal illness.

TYPES OF DEATH

This is my death ... and it will profit me to understand it.

Anne Sexton, *The Death Notebooks*, 1974

Traditional ways of deciding what type of death has occurred use such categories as accidental, suicide, homicide, and death by natural causes. Physicians have further categorized death according to the disease that was the primary cause, while carrying out epidemiological studies. The authors looked for other existing and accepted descriptors that are useful. Two of those categories are expected death and sudden death.

Expected Death

The term *expected death*, which is in limited use, refers to the dying or terminal patient. When the College of Physicians and Surgeons of Manitoba (Canada), The Winnipeg Community and Long Term Care Authority, and others created guidelines to ensure continuity of care of the terminally ill, they wrote "Arrangements for Expected Death at Home-108" (www.umanitoba.ca/colleges/cps/Guidelines_and_Statements/108.html).

Eisenberg and Mengert (2001), in their article "Cardiac Resuscitation," use the term when referring to the quandary facing an emergency medical team treating a patient who has a bad heart and is expected to die but is resuscitated regardless of his or her family's wishes.

More than 90 per cent of Americans will die from a protracted life-threatening illness, according to Linda Emanuel and colleagues (1999) in their textbook *Education for Physicians on End-of-life Care*. Patients with cancer suffer a steady decline and a brief terminal time period. Those with illnesses such as emphysema and Alzheimer's experience a slow decline, with occasional medical emergencies, ending in sudden death. When the authors use the term *expected death*, they refer to the terminal phase only.

Education for Physicians on End-of-Life Care refers to expected death at various points in the curriculum, including in Module 12, "Last Hours of Living." The curriculum recommends, for example, that as expected death approaches, the medical team clarify the goals of care and the futility of interventions aimed at prolonging life (Emanuel et al., 1999).

Slow codes are a controversial way of responding to expected deaths. These codes are "cardiopulmonary resuscitative efforts, which involve a deliberate decision not to attempt aggressively to bring a patient back to life" (Gazelle, 1998b, 467). Although considered unethical by many, medical teams use them for patients with dementia, in comas, or in advanced terminal illnesses. Such patients, who are expected to die, have left no DNR orders or wishes about how they want to die (Gazelle, 1998a). (A discussion of this subject, including pros and cons, appears in Gazelle, 1998b.)

When physicians expect a death, the patient is usually suffering from a condition caused by overwhelming trauma or has an illness for which treatment is no longer possible. Aggressive full codes and invasive procedures may no longer be meaningful medically and may appear futile. Palliative care and hospice are meaningful choices at these times.

Sudden, or Unexpected, Death

Sudden death, defined by Sherwin Nuland, is an "unexpected death within a few hours of onset of symptoms in persons neither hospitalized nor homebound" (Nuland, 1995: 18). Sudden death can be accidental, violent, or an acute catastrophic medical death, such as a myocardial infarction or massive stroke. Less than 10 per cent of Americans will die from an unexpected and sudden death according to Emanuel et al. (1999) in *Education for Physicians on End-of-Life Care*.

A sudden death, then, is unexpected. Unless a person who dies in this way had the foresight to discuss her wishes with her family or pre-arrange a funeral, her family and the attending medical staff must decide what to do with her body.

In an accidental death, caused, for example, by drowning, a car accident, accidental shooting, or domestic accident, family members may suffer not just the shock of the incident but also guilt and shame about what they might have done differently. A patient of JS, who had been recently divorced and was drinking heavily, had an argument with her son. Extremely angry, her son sped away on his motorcycle. He lost control of the bike, crashed, and died from neck trauma. His mother experienced a deep sense of guilt. She questioned all that happened: "What if I hadn't argued with my son? Why didn't I tell him I loved him? Why didn't I say goodbye before he left? Why did I get divorced?" Because of her guilt, she had a very difficult time dealing with her son's accidental death.

If a violent death occurs in a war, the family, though mournful, may feel pride in the loved one, who served the country and died for a cause. Recognition and support can also lend meaning and ease the pain of loss in extraordinary situations. After thousands of innocent people died unexpectedly and violently when two airplanes crashed into the World Trade Towers in New York City on September 11, 2001, many Americans made financial contributions in order to help the families of the victims. The policemen and firemen who gave up their lives and risked their personal safety to save others were eulogized.

When a violent death is random, as it is in a drive-by shooting, the shock is intense and sudden. The anger goes deep, especially if the perpetrator is not found. In 1996, a stranger abducted nine-year-old Amber Hagerman, who was living in Arlington, Texas. Her killer was never found. The community, which continues to grieve for her, holds a vigil each year on the anniversary of her death.

In medical sudden death, which occurs when, for example, a child dies of asthma or an adult of a heart attack or stroke, family members may feel guilt over not intervening earlier. This is also true when a family member dies suddenly as a result of alcohol or drug abuse. George McGovern was devastated when his beloved daughter Terry froze to death in a snowbank after an evening of heavy drinking. In his book *Terry* (McGovern, 1996), he asked himself what he could have done differently to prevent her death or her alcoholism.

Several studies have found sudden, unexpected death results in a more difficult bereavement, although this is not always the case (Lundin, 1984). Coping is often easier when the person who died suddenly is elderly. The sudden death of a young person is always traumatic (Parkes, 1998). Following a sudden death, especially that of a child, the family members should be allowed to hold or touch the deceased, whenever possible (Rutkowski, 2002).

This chapter confirms that medical education has mostly ignored end-of-life care, although compelling reasons exist for preparing physicians to help the dying and their families, as well as themselves.

2

Stages of Dying

It is also the recognition that the *real* event taking place at the end of our life is our death, not the attempts to prevent it.
  Sherwin Nuland, *How We Die: Reflections on Life's Final Chapter*, 1994

SOME EXISTING THEORIES OF DYING

Beginning in the 1960s, physicians and other theorists began to develop models of death and dying. The most popular is probably Elisabeth Kübler-Ross's theory. Charles Corr, Barney Glaser, Anselm Straus, and Robert Buckman developed other theories. These theorists helped bring the concept of death and dying to the public and physicians' attention (Copp, 1998).

Elisabeth Kübler-Ross's Five-Stage Theory

In her pivotal 1969 book *On Death and Dying*, Elisabeth Kübler-Ross described the five stages a person goes through when dealing with death: denial, anger, bargaining, depression, and acceptance (Kübler-Ross, 1969). When in denial, the dying person attempts to refute or escape the death sentence. The person then goes on to experience anger, often asking repeatedly, "Why me?" The dying person may direct this rage and resentment toward members of the family and medical professionals. In the third stage, bargaining, the dying person attempts to make some type of private deal with fate or God. Eventually the person becomes depressed and mournful. In the final state, acceptance, the patient comes to terms with death. These five stages help the physician understand how patients' feelings change over time. In reality, the stages do not necessarily appear in the above order and do not always end in acceptance.

When JS completed her medical training, she repaid her student loan by working in a prison. Each month she routinely saw the prisoners with chronic illnesses. Mike S., 48, had a lung tumor on his x-ray. He denied this fact adamantly and was enraged at JS, whom he accused of incompetence. This prisoner later had a seizure, as his lung cancer had metastasized to his brain. He was flown to the prison hospital, where JS visited him. By then, having accepted his illness, his calmer, gentler self had emerged. He went through the stages of denial, anger, and acceptance. Knowing that his anger and rage were common reactions to a terminal diagnosis, JS was not put off or hurt and was able to care for the man.

B.G. Glaser and A.L. Straus's Context of Awareness Theory

B.G. Glaser and A.L. Strauss used a sociological approach to develop their model of dying (Glaser and Straus, 1965, Copp, 1998). They collected data from four hospitals in the San Francisco Bay area, interviewing hospital staff and patients with life-threatening illnesses. They described four contexts of awareness among hospital staffs and patients: closed awareness, suspicion awareness, mutual pretense awareness, and open awareness.

In closed awareness, the doctors and nurses and other staff did not discuss the future, circumvented disclosure of the illness, and kept medical conversations to a minimum. For example, JS treated an elderly Buddhist, Lon N. He did not speak English, so the family translated English into Vietnamese for him. His family did not tell him he was dying, as JS requested, because doing so went against their value system. JS will never know if he died peacefully, unaware of his impending death.

Suspicion awareness is an unstable situation that occurs when patients begin to suspect that they are dying and that the staff will not tell them this. Patients may sneak a look at their chart or ask the staff directly. The staff prevents such patients from knowing the truth by controlling their facial expressions and their mannerisms and reactions.

The daughter of Rosa S., an early Alzheimer's patient in her seventies, did not want her mother to know she had this terminal illness. Even when Rosa asked the nursing home staff directly, no one would tell her the diagnosis. Glaser and Straus (1965) believe that suspicion awareness puts a great psychological strain on families, the staff, and the patient.

Mutual pretense awareness occurs when both patient and staff know the patient is dying but no one will discuss the situation. Marty T., who had metastatic colon cancer, knew that his chemotherapy was failing but believed that if he gave up he would disappoint the medical staff, which had fought so hard for him. The medical staff respected Marty's courage. None of them wanted to tell him his treatment was failing, fearing he would lose hope and feel that his suffering had been in vain. Marty died alone because he could not discuss his fears with the staff. The situation of mutual pretense awareness imposes stress on all involved, as is apparent in Marty's story.

When both the patient and staff acknowledge that the patient is dying, there is open awareness. Open awareness has its own uncertainties and ambiguities, especially when the patient's style of dying conflicts with the staff's. Although Fred M. had end-stage AIDS in 1985, he wanted everything done to help him live. He had early HIV dementia, a low CD4 count, fevers, and many hospitalizations due to mycobacterium avian sepsis. While the nursing staff wanted him in hospice, he wanted all available treatments. In the end, he got what he wanted. Because the life-saving "cocktail" existed by then, Fred is alive and well today thanks to the "cocktail."

Robert Buckman's Three-Stage Model

Robert Buckman (1998) developed a three-stage model of death and dying. His theory is based on two main principles:

1 Patients who face death exhibit a mixture of reactions that are characteristic of the patient, not of the diagnosis or stage of the dying process.
2 Patients progress emotionally because they resolve emotions, not because they feel different emotions.

While in the initial stage in this model, facing the threat of death, the patient's emotions may include fear, anxiety, shock, disbelief, anger, denial, guilt, humor, hope, despair, or bargaining. The emotions are unique to the patient and his life history. No two patients react alike when they are told that they could die. Mike Z., 86, had always been active in his Jewish community. Although he had been forced to immigrate twice and his life had been difficult, he was a positive person. After he fractured his hip, he became completely dependent on others. Because he loathed being dependent, he hoped for death, frequently asking. "Is it over yet?" He viewed death as his escape from mental and physical anguish.

The second stage is the chronic stage or the stage of being ill. In this stage the patient resolves any of the elements of the initial stage that are resolvable. Emotions diminish in intensity and become almost monotone. Depression is common in this stage. Sister Abby, a devout Catholic nun who believed she was married to Jesus, prayed daily to God. Angry with God for abandoning her when she developed breast cancer, she became very depressed. She asked, "How could God do this to me?"

During acceptance, the final stage of this model, patients accept death. A few days before her death, Sister Abby seemed at peace. She stated that she was ready to meet her Maker and looked forward to death so that she could be with God. While acceptance brings peace, as it did to Sister Abby, acceptance is not an essential stage, provided the patient is making normal decisions, communicating well, and is not distressed.

C.A. Corr's Task-Based Approach to Dying

C.A. Corr (1992, 1998) believes that individuals have four primary tasks when coping with dying: the physical, the psychological, the social, and the spiritual. Corr holds that there is no right way to cope with dying and that the act of dying is not confined to the individual. All of those involved are affected, including nurses and doctors.

Physical tasks address satisfying bodily needs and minimizing physical distress in ways that are consistent with personal values. For instance, John G., a Buddhist, wanted to die alone and in a quiet place. This was his way of relaxing his body.

Psychological tasks involve maximizing psychological security, autonomy, and richness of living. Following his beliefs, John wrote out his own funeral service and arranged for care of his body. He meditated daily to help maintain mental calmness.

Social tasks include sustaining and enhancing significant interpersonal attachments and addressing the social implications of dying.

John told his family and friends of his impending death and arranged for care of a beloved dog.

When attending to spiritual tasks, the patient identifies, develops and reaffirms sources of spiritual energy, thereby fostering hope. John re-examined his beliefs in Buddhism and was more at peace as a result.

> Death belongs to life as birth does. The walk is in the raising of the foot as in the laying of it down.
>
> Rabindranath Tagore, 1985

Jan Swanson's and Alan Cooper's Six Stages of Dying

As physicians treat the patient and their significant others before and after death, they often see many sides of the process of dying that only clergy and families witness. This can be a gift or a burden, depending upon how doctors handle the demands involved.

As they witness the process of dying, physicians face various stages related to their patients' deaths. Based on their observations in provision of patient care and review of the literature, the authors have identified six stages: recognition, the process of dying, the moment of death, the departure of the spirit or life force, terminal care of the body, and dealing with grief.

These stages serve as a heuristic device to organize elements of the dying process that the physician encounters at various times. The authors realize that research will determine whether this is a useful model or not.

The first stage, recognition, is similar to the stage that Buckman labels facing the threat of death. While Buckman focuses on the patient's perspective, the authors also consider what the physician and other caregivers might witness and the last three stages they discuss occur after the person has died. The authors' stages are a conceptualization intended to help physicians identify the needs of patients and their loved ones before and after death. The authors explain the spiritual, physical, emotional, and social needs of those affected, including the patient, his or her family, friends and caregivers, such as nurses and physicians.

Like Corr, the authors believe that the act of dying is not confined to the individual but affects all involved. The authors also agree with Corr's belief that there is no right way to die and that whenever possible patients should be able to die in a way that suits them. The authors also acknowledge that the concept of open awareness, as described by Glaser and Strauss, helps to bring about a peaceful death.

While the primary perspective of the authors is that of the physician, three of their stages also refer to the patient's experience and decisions to be made. The authors' view is complementary to a subjective perspective like Buckman's. The authors are not suggesting that the physician's perspective is superior to that of the patient but hope their stages will prove useful in a different way.

RECOGNITION

The patient recognizes, for a first moment, that life is approaching its end and realizes that death will occur in weeks, months, or a year, rather than in some very distant future. A physician's words, the patient's awareness of a problem, or a spiritual awakening may create the moment of awareness in a patient. A person who is unaware of his mortality may be more careless than a person who understands his days as finite. Such patients may modify goals and relationships with loved ones.

The words, or even the expression, of a doctor can spark recognition of life-threatening illness. Evan Handler, author of *Time on Fire* (1996), and John Gunther, author of *Death Be Not Proud* (1949), describe how the behaviour and expressions of their doctors revealed to them that they or a relative had a life-threatening illness.

Handler writes: "I think that was the first time I ever felt scared in a doctor's office. Because the doctor seemed concerned, about something in particular, and finding evidence of what he was concerned about. Dread is what I really felt. A sudden, short, deep stab of dread" (Handler, 1996:16).

The looks on the doctors' faces told Gunther his teenage son was dying. He wrote, "I cannot explain this except by saying that I saw it on the faces of the three doctors, particularly Kahn's. I never met this good doctor again, but I will never forget the way he kept his face averted while he talked, then another glimpse of his blank, averted face as he said goodbye, dark with all that he was sparing us, all that he knew would happen to Johnny, and that I didn't know and Frances didn't know and that neither of us should know for as long as possible" (Gunther, 1949:21). Because what doctors say and how they say it profoundly affects patients and their families, the authors suggest that physicians should pause and plan what they say as carefully as they make a diagnosis, perform a procedure, or deliver a baby.

Recognition of death is difficult for all involved. Patients may learn for the first time the name of an illness they knew nothing about. They may ask: "What is this illness? What did I do to get this? Will my children have this disease? What treatment is available to me? How long will I live? Will I suffer with this disease? Who should treat me and where should I be treated?"

Patients may also ask questions that relate to their families and finances: "Who will care for my family when I am sick or if I should die? Can I afford this medical care?" or "What will happen to my job?" or "How will I care for myself?" For example, a woman with breast cancer must learn what kind of breast cancer she has and decide who will operate on her and who will treat her medically. Will she have a mastectomy, a mastectomy and reconstruction, or a lumpectomy? Should she have chemotherapy before surgery and both radiation and chemotherapy following? Should she have genetic testing or not? Should her children have genetic testing? She must deal with a changing body image and the prospect of death. Overwhelmed as she is, her health care providers and family are probably telling her to hurry in making her decisions. The woman who finds out she has breast cancer is at an important fork in the road. A wrong decision may result in death.

Physicians and health professionals can help patients at this first stage by being aware of the deep impact their diagnosis has on patients and their families. Physicians can clearly describe illness and treatment to patients in compassionate words, allowing them time to ask questions. Doctors should realize that what is routine to them may be the worst moment in a patient's life (Kastenbaum and Kastenbaum, 1989).

Recognition of mortality, though an internal experience for patients, will manifest itself in the types of questions they ask and in the emotional states that may accompany this stage. Recognition will often compete with denial in the early stages of a life-threatening illness. Denial can serve as a protective cushioning, so that patients may show little interest in talking about how serious their prognosis is. However, at some point, awareness of the illness becomes inescapable; patients begin to acknowledge more clearly what has become obvious to others. Emotions at this point include anxiety, anger, and despair, just as they do in Buckman's *facing the threat of death* stage. Patients experience intense and sometimes shifting emotional states, depending on their personalities. They may let others know what they are feeling and thinking in verbal and non-verbal communications with physicians and nurses. Patients will also ask questions that reveal their concerns, as their awareness of mortality grows.

Recognition may even be necessary to provide appropriate health care to the dying patient. Physicians have a duty to inform patients that they are dying. As the authors will discuss later, doctors need to be compassionate while performing this duty. They should talk to their patients in a way that makes them as comfortable as possible and only when they are ready to do so (Stolick, 2002).

> The long habit of living indisposeth us for dying.
> Sir Thomas Browne (1605–1682), *Hydriotaphia and The Garden of Cyprus*

THE PROCESS OF DYING

During this stage, the body is deteriorating. This can occur quickly when there is an accident or unusual circumstance. A patient of JS, who had an infected breast implant, suddenly became septic. Within hours her renal function was impaired so that her potassium level was elevated. She went into ventricular tachycardia and briefly lost consciousness. Quick resuscitation brought her back. That patient remembers the staff calling her name while she was unconscious, as if they were calling her back to life.

Dying may also occur slowly, as it does when patients have AIDS, cancer, or heart disease. Cancer slowly invades surrounding organs and causes them to malfunction and shut down, while advanced HIV allows illnesses such as an opportunistic infection to invade until the body shuts down.

Walt Swanson, the father of JS, had smoked three packs of cigarettes daily since adolescence. The cigarettes slowly began to take a toll on his health, so that when he was 49 he developed lung cancer. The cancer was found early and he had one lung removed in surgery. He quit cigarettes, lost weight, and exercised. He even published two books and wrote a play. However, his heart and lung did not maintain their original vigor. When JS was a medical student in Lansing, she noticed that Walt was frequently short of breath and often had what she thought were angina attacks. JS would constantly run the CPR resuscitation protocol through her mind when he visited; she was worried he would suffer cardiac arrest and wanted to be there for him. Walt died of cardiac arrest in late October 1982, when he was 65 years old. His autopsy showed diffuse coronary artery disease and pulmonary hypertension. Shortly before his death, Walt told JS that he thought that he began dying when he developed lung cancer.

When treating patients with HIV or another life-threatening condition, JS understands that outward appearances are not reliable indicators of health or sickness. A patient of JS, an upbeat man is his fifties, was looking great, although his T-cell count was below 20. One day she noticed that he was dragging a leg, the first sign of multifocal leukoencephalopathy. He gradually became unable to walk. She explained to him that his illness had no known effective treatments at the time. At this point, he decided to go on hospice. As time wore on, he was less able to care for himself and became comatose just before he died.

Another AIDS patient, whose had a conservative religious background, found it difficult to face the fact that he had AIDS, since the way he had acquired the disease involved activities that his religion and background opposed. When he was close to dying, JS told the patient that he could continue treatment, be a no code, or be in hospice. He was furious with her, telling her she was frightening him. She felt as if she was only a foot tall and was frustrated because she wanted him to know all his options. Thinking back, JS wishes she had asked the patient how much information he wanted to know about his illness at that point or whether there was a family member that he wanted her to talk to on his behalf. This patient had a right to know the information being offered but needed to know it on his own terms.

When deterioration in health occurs, patients need to decide what treatment, if any, they will have. They need to decide who will have their medical power of attorney, whether they want to sign a DNR order, and whether or not to be in hospice. They need to recognize that they will have to deal with a failing body, a deteriorating physical appearance, and the accompanying fear. Physicians can help such patients by giving them options and arranging for care and medicine. Physicians can let them know what financial and spiritual support exists in the community. They can also listen to them and their families.

During the process of dying the patient experiences a transition from good health to an awareness that the body is failing. It is a time of adjustment, planning, and reconciliation.

> Dying is a wild night and a new road.
>
> Emily Dickinson (1830-1886)

THE MOMENT OF DEATH

This occurs when the life force leaves the body. The state is almost impossible to describe, since the experts – those who have died – are not here to describe dying. The authors believe that Gunther offers one of the most touching descriptions, when describing the passing of his son. In *Death Be Not Proud*, Gunther wrote:

Three great quivering gasps came out of him. He had color just before; he had some final essential spark of animation; he was still fighting. But now these shatteringly deep breaths, arising from somewhere so deep down that his whole body shook and trembled, told us their irrevocable message. Johnny died at 11:02 PM. Frances reached for him through the ugly, transparent, raincoat-like curtain of the oxygen machine. I felt his arms, cupping my hands around them, and the warmth gradually left them, receding very slowly upward from his hands. For a long time some warmth remained. Then little by little the life-color left his face, his lips became blue, and his hands were cold. What is life? It departs covertly. Like a thief, Death took him. (Gunther, 1949:16)

One evening JS visited a minister, Charlie B., who was in the hospital dying of lung cancer and was aware that he would die that night. His heart was racing and he had severe, laboured respirations. His last concern was his family's well being, so he paid some bills when his daughter handed him some checks. After he had paid the last bill, his eyes turned upward and he died. His body was spiritless. Only a few minutes before, it had contained a man with a purpose.

Martin R., a 48-year-old physician, participated in the authors' study. He had a near-death experience while living with AIDS. When asked what happens when a person dies, he replied, "I just don't know. My experience was simply an awareness that I might not awaken. I was totally clear that in any event I would be dead. There was more a sense of curiosity than anything else. There was no white light, no beckoning tunnels, just quiet." (Martin has since died from complications of AIDS.)

The moment of death is a major life event. Because no one really knows what happens, almost everyone is frightened. Like birth, death is an exit from one world into another. Physicians can help patients deal with their fear by doing everything possible to ensure that they are pain-free, where they want to be when they die, and not alone.

> Because I could not stop for Death,
> He kindly stopped for me.
>
> Emily Dickinson

QUESTIONS FOR HEALTH CARE PROFESSIONALS

What do you believe happens to a person at the moment of death?

SAMPLE ANSWER: I think people feel their life ebb slowly away as they become weaker and weaker and return to their original oneness with the universe.

YOUR ANSWER:

The Departure of the Spirit or Life Force

JS has watched many patients die. She is aware, then, that a patient will have a personality and feel warm to the touch at one moment, then appear motionless and spiritless the next. What happened to the spirit?

Pastor Michael Pozar, who is director of Lutheran AIDS Network in San Francisco, wrote for the authors' study why he believed people need a concept of what happens to them when they die. "Jung felt that the important thing was that a person have a clear concept of an afterlife (or absence thereof) and that it is the people with no clear concept who are the most troubled in dying."

Several of those who participated in the authors' study provided the following thoughts on what happens to the spirit at the moment of death: Reverend Pat Enkyo O'Hara, a Buddhist, writes, "They drop their physical husk. They become dead: they are no longer understandable to the living. The transformation into Oneness, the Unborn of the One Body – the Universe itself."

Payam Maveddat, a Baha'i', explains his beliefs: "Concerning the future life, what the Baha'u'llah (the founder of faith) says is that the soul will continue to ascend through many worlds. What those worlds are and what their nature is we cannot know. The same way that the child in the matrix cannot know this world, so we cannot know what the other world is going to be." A 43-year-old addiction-ologist shares her view: "I hope their soul goes to heaven. I'm pretty sure their bodies become fertilizer."

Life is a great surprise. I do not see why death should not be an even greater one.

Vladimir Nabokov, *Pale Fire*, 1989

QUESTIONS FOR HEALTH CARE PROFESSIONALS

What do you believe happens to the spirit or soul, if anything, when you die? How does this affect your care of patients?

SAMPLE ANSWER: No one knows for sure. We at least remain in the universe as matter. I believe we are reincarnated to deal with our weaknesses. For instance, if we are prejudiced against a particular sex or race, we will be reborn as a member of that group. Because our spirit lives on, I believe that bodies need to be treated with respect.

YOUR ANSWER:

TERMINAL CARE OF THE BODY

The care of the body starts at the moment of death and continues through the funeral until its final disposition. Nurses, doctors, and loved ones must decide what will happen to the bodies of those who die. Should they be left in the room for a while, sent to the family's home, buried, cremated, be disposed of immediately or after some specified period of time? Should there be a wake? Dying patients find all these matters a great concern. Ryan White, who died of AIDS, was much less anxious about dying after he saw the cemetery where he would be buried. Elisabeth Kübler-Ross wrote of a patient who was afraid of dying because she believed that if she were buried, her body would be eaten by worms. She was relieved to learn about cremation. Some people believe they cannot go to heaven or to their final spiritual resting place if their body is not handled correctly.

Physicians can have some control in these matters. When JS was a supervising intern, a student wanted to practise intubation on a patient who had just died. JS, who found this very upsetting, refused permission. The medical student went over her head, appealing to the doctor in charge. He agreed to the intubation, because he felt it would help future patients. JS still feels the doctor and intern failed to respect the dead patient, since interns can practise intubation during an anesthesia rotation. She had been taught respect of the dead while in medical school at Michigan State University. The instructor in charge of the school's anatomy lab told the medical students that cadavers were people who had graciously donated their bodies so students could become better doctors. The students were not allowed to laugh or use morbid humor; if they did, they were expelled from the school.

If a family member is not treated with respect, the family may be upset. The following statements are from the authors' study. Bill G., whose brother died at 47 of AIDS at the Veterans Administration Hospital, was upset when the nurses refused to enter the room after his brother's death and when they told him that the body must be removed from the hospital as soon as possible.

An 81-year-old woman, Elsie A., when discussing how her husband's body was handled, wrote: "My husband was taken to the morgue for cremation. This was around Christmas. The reception desk had me sign for a Gala Christmas bag. Upon opening it, I found a plastic box with his ashes." What a thoughtless act toward the woman and her dead husband! There is no reason that a body should ever be treated without respect and dignity.

Each religion has its own sets of rules and rituals that apply to the body after death. The authors have selected descriptions from three religious traditions from their study. Rabbi Kenneth Roseman of Dallas, who frowns on cremation, suggests burials as soon as possible after death, usually within 24–36 hours. He believes that healing does not begin until after the funeral.

Payam Maveddat, a member of the Baha'i' faith, states that according to Baha'i' writings: "The body must not be transported more than an hour's journey from the place of death. Before transport, the body should be carefully washed and placed in a shroud of white cloth, preferably silk. Finally, the person should be buried within 24 hours of the time of death."

Reverend Rodney de Martini writes, "In the Catholic tradition the body must be treated with reverence, perhaps anointed and bathed after death by family or friends before it is entrusted to the mortuary. Cremation and embalming are seen as acceptable but limited to personal or family decisions."

In summary, most religious creeds have a specified ceremony or funeral service. In any case, handling a body with respect and dignity requires just a small effort. Caring for the body is the doctor's final way to respect the deceased and comfort those who remain.

> For dust thou art, and unto dust shalt thou return.
>
> Genesis 3:19

QUESTIONS FOR HEALTH CARE PROFESSIONALS

Upon your death, how would you want your body handled?

SAMPLE ANSWER: I would not want medical students to practise intubation on me. I would not want to leave the place I died in a plastic body bag. I would want to be covered with a sheet. I would want to be an organ donor and would like to have my ashes scattered on the ocean, which would remind me that I am but a small part of the universe. I would also like to have a memorial service.

YOUR ANSWER:

DEALING WITH GRIEF

Grief is a normal process. Dying patients grieve the loss of health and function and the impending loss of life, while family and friends feel anticipatory grief. JS once imagined how she would respond if told she had cancer. She realized that she would have to say goodbye not only to her family, friends, and animals, but also to the seasons, daily activities, sunlight, trees, and flowers. She could imagine the sense of deep loss she would feel almost immediately.

According to Robert and Bernice Kastenbaum, authors of *The Encyclopedia of Death* (1989), mourning is not the same as grief. Mourning is a patterned ritual, which depends upon religious and cultural traditions. A person can mourn without feeling grief and feel grief without mourning.

People experience grief in response to loss. Normal or uncomplicated grief is a healthy response to losses of all sorts, including the loss of a job, a divorce, and the death of a child or spouse. Patients and caretakers also experience grief when faced with terminal illness. In fact, anticipatory grief may help a family member who has begun to anticipate life alone and progressed from denying the seriousness of the illness to preparing for the future (Zeitlin, 2001).

Common feelings associated with normal grief include sadness, anxiety, anger, and relief. Common physical sensations include lack of energy, tightness in the throat, and a feeling of unreality. Common thoughts that occur in the early stages of grief include confusion, obsession with thoughts of the departed, and even hallucinations. The latter are common, transient, and usually only occur within a few weeks of the death (Worden, 2002).

Bereavement has its own risks, as it is associated with higher rates of health problems, depression, drug and alcohol problems, suicide, and mortality (Penson et al., 2002, Schaefer et al., 1995). A person who experiences complicated grief may be at greater risk for morbidity due to cancer, hypertension, cardiac events, and depression than a person who experiences simple grief. (See Prigerson and Jacobs, 2001 for many references on these topics.)

Grief becomes complicated as the grief reaction becomes more intense, lasts longer, and affects physical and emotional health. Examples of complicated grief reactions are chronic grief, which lasts for over a year unabated; delayed grief, which is postponed or suppressed; exaggerated grief, which results in self-destructive behaviour; and masked grief, which is not experienced directly,

appearing instead as a medical complaint such as pain or unex-
plained depression (von Gunten et al., 2000). Lacking a completely
clear definition, complicated grief is usually associated with psychiatric sequelae, such as major depression and substance abuse
(Penson et al., 2002).

In *Grief Counseling and Grief Therapy*, J. William Worden (2002)
identified the following mediators as very likely to influence the intensity of the grief reaction and the course grief was likely to take.

Mediator 1: Who the Person Was

The relationship to the deceased: A person will grieve a distant
cousin or a rarely seen grandparent in a different way than he will
grieve for his beloved spouse, his child, a life-long companion,
or a grandparent who had raised him. A psychotherapy patient
of Alan Cooper (referred to hereafter as AC) became clinically
depressed after his favourite grandmother died. Her love for him
had always been certain, while his family was cold and abusive.

Mediator 2: The Nature of the Attachment

The strength of the attachment: One of AC's patients went
through a difficult time when her elderly mother was killed in a
car accident. The patient had always depended on her mother to
tell her what to do and think and even how to raise her child. In a
matter of hours after the death, the woman found herself forced
to make decisions that would have been inconceivable before her
mother died. Although the daughter's suffering was intense, during the months following the death she could see that her loss
clearly marked the beginning of her adulthood.

Ambivalence in the relationship: A study by Colin Parkes and
Robert Weiss, authors of *Recovery From Bereavement* (1983),
identified eight risk factors that predicted the extent of support
family members need after the death of a loved one. Although
the results of the study, which was done at London's St. Christopher's Hospice, may not generalize to all populations, two factors
are relevant to the authors' discussion: high anger and high self-
reproach. A respected writer on grief counselling, Worden noted
that when negative feelings exist in almost equal proportion to
positive feelings, the grieving process will almost always be difficult (1991).

Another of AC's patients had a very difficult time allowing herself to grieve when her mother died after a long battle with heart disease. Whenever she began to miss her mother, she felt guilty that she had not led the life her mother had expected of her. For example, she was not actively involved in her mother's fundamentalist church. Although she had not wanted to be, she still felt guilty. In psychotherapy, she had to deal with her right to lead her own life before she could grieve her mother's loss in a healthy way.

Mediator 3: Mode of Death

The circumstances of death and whether it was preventable: Family members may worry about whether they took their loved one to a physician soon enough, the physician was the right physician, or the hospital was the right hospital. Guilt is a very powerful emotion. They may worry about whether or not they should have signed permission to do surgery and whether they spent enough time with their loved one prior to death. AC counselled a married couple where the wife had recently lost her father, whom her husband considered a good friend as well as a father-in-law. The husband felt guilty, because he believed that if he had spent nearly every waking minute with his father-in- law, he could have boosted his will to live and perhaps saved his life. The wife, who was not that close to her formerly neglectful father, did not agree that her husband was responsible for keeping her father alive. She felt let down, because her husband was away from home so much while caring for her father.

The suddenness of death: How survivors grieve may depend on whether the person they lost died from natural causes, in an accident, or as a result of suicide or a homicide. How well family members cope also depends on how much notice they have about a death.

AC's father became increasingly disabled over several months, so that during one visit he was even unable to recognize AC. As a result, AC felt as if he had lost his father long before he died. His actual death came as a relief to AC and the family.

The manner of death notification: The manner in which physicians tell families that one of their members has died can affect their grief. Below, three individuals who participated in the authors' study describe how they learned about the death of a relative. They also suggest what the physicians involved could have done to make the experience easier.

- An 81-year-old woman, Elsie A., remembered that someone from her husband's nursing home called to say he had died shortly after she had visited him. She said she never heard from his doctor, adding bitterly that she had received his bill.
- Juan M. described the death of his father from cirrhosis of the liver: "I was informed by phone by relatives who were at his side. The doctor spoke Spanish and was able to convey to my mother that his condition was deteriorating. She felt very relieved to know what was actually happening. When my father lost brain activity, my mother was consulted to let her know what options were available to her."
- Johnny N. described the death of his mother from stroke and heart disease: "I was there when she took her last breath. No physician can make a dying experience better for anyone, other than providing support. I do believe the physician is responsible to give full knowledge to the family of what is occurring at the time it is occurring."

Mediator 4: Historical Antecedents
How well a person coped with previous loss: Everyone has a loss history, which includes the deaths of family, friends, and even pets. This history also includes divorces, geographical moves, and loss of possessions. How well a person is prepared and able to cope with these losses has a significant effect on response to future loss. A patient of AC, whose mother had died, was preparing to move in with her emotionally volatile sister. She hoped that they could help each other deal with the loss. Before she completed the move, her sister committed suicide, creating even greater loss.

Mediator 5: Personality Variables
The personality and coping patterns of the grieving person, their ability to express emotions, seek, and receive help: According to Worden and other sources people with certain personalities or problems will experience significant difficulty grieving the loss of a loved one. They include highly dependent people, narcissistic personalities, borderline personalities, people coping with depres-

sion or bipolar illness, and very anxious people or very isolated people. One patient told AC that he coped with his father's death by drinking heavily for months. Although this only postponed his grieving, he wasn't willing to give up the alcohol until his high level of drinking became apparent to everyone.

The person's general health and lifestyle practises: A patient of JS became very concerned when she experienced chest pains shortly after her husband died from a myocardial infarction. Her physician at the time ruled out cardiovascular problems and recommended she find a counsellor. Somatic complaints and increased illness may signify that a person is unable to grieve or adjust to a loss.

Radical changes in lifestyle following a death may also be a sign of unresolved grief. Patients responding to loss may abuse alcohol or drugs, work excessively hard, or become addictive in other ways. They are putting the grieving process on hold.

Mediator 6: Social Variables

The strength and nature of the support system including cultural and religious beliefs: Patients who had joined grief support groups reported to the authors that they were very helpful. Individual grief counselling sessions can also provide real support, particularly when a patient's grief is complicated by complex emotions and unfinished business. *The Grief Recovery Handbook*, by John James and Russell Friedman (1998), is an excellent resource for those in any stage of grief recovery. James and Friedman recommend that recovering people avoid isolation and find partners to help them grieve. Such partners should have experienced intense emotional loss in their lives, although they need not have suffered a similar loss. Partners may be family members, co-workers, friends, or fellow church members. Partners can help those grieving examine incomplete emotional relationships, make amends, offer forgiveness, and begin to move beyond loss.

Unhelpful partners fear the feelings of the grieving, according to James and Friedman. These partners tend to refuse to discuss death, change the subject when it comes up, or don't know what to say. They may also intellectualize or tell the grieving person not to be angry with God. These well-meaning but unhelpful people encourage those grieving to stay busy, bury their feelings, replace their loss, or "just give it time." Partners provide real help only

when they tolerate and accept complex, intense, and even contradictory feelings, so that those grieving can express their emotions
without fear of judgment. JS cried for three days after her father
died. Everyone was upset by her behaviour and strong emotional
reaction. Yet only after those three days could JS begin to lead her
life again.

Mediator 7: Concurrent Stresses

Pressures from other sources: Certain changes and disruptions,
such as moves, job changes, and financial crises, which often follow a death, especially the death of a life partner or spouse, are
associated with depression (Worden, 1996).

Grief is not a disease; it is a normal healing process that temporarily impairs function. Grief is necessary to allow healthy functioning
to return and for emotional growth to continue. Worden identified
four tasks family and friends need to undertake in order to complete
the grieving process:

Task 1: Accept the reality of the loss.
Come to terms with the fact that the loved one is gone forever.
Task 2: Work through the pain of grief.
Feel the pain of the loss. Do not avoid reminders of the dead, turn
to alcohol and drugs, work too hard, or travel from place to place.
Task 3: Adjust to an environment in which the deceased is missing.
The first year after a death is hard for a partner who is left to live,
raise children, and manage a home and finances alone. In addition
to adjusting to external events, which requires the development of
new skills and roles, the grieving person must also adjust internally, because, as Worden points out, death also affects the definition of self and self esteem. A widowed person finds it increasingly
difficult to define himself or herself in relation to the deceased.
Task 4: Emotionally relocate the deceased and move on with life.
Those grieving never forget those they lose, but eventually they
create in their thoughts and memories a new relationship, so they
can reinvest in life. They then realize that there are new people to
love. This long-term process may take at least a year. According
to Worden, when the grieving person is able to think about the
deceased without pain or crying and has regained an interest in
life, grieving may come to an end. One of AC's patients, who lost

his wife of 30 years, did not believe that he could undertake this task, since his grief was so profound. He believed his thoughts and feelings would continue to focus almost entirely on his wife. As the months went by, however, he became increasingly involved in various activities and developed stronger relationships with his friends. (Worden, 2000)

HELPING THE FAMILY WITH GRIEF

What can the physician do for the family after the death of the patient to help this healing process? Often the family does not hear from the doctor, who may be avoiding his own grief over the loss of the patient, feeling guilty about the death, or fearing the family's upset feelings (Holland, 2002).

Physicians may wonder if they should call or write a note to the family. They may find that a brief telephone call or a note offering reassurance or recalling a positive story about the deceased can be very comforting (Holland, 2002). Susanna Bedell and her colleagues (2001) recommend writing a condolence letter with these elements:

- A direct expression of sorrow about the death
- A personal memory of the patient and something about the patient's family or work
- Specific references to achievement at work, devotion to family, courage during the illness, or the patient's character
- State that it was a privilege to have participated in the patient's care (1163).

Should physicians attend the funeral? Obviously, this is often impossible, but if attending the funeral will help doctors deal with their own grief at losing patients with whom they became particularly close, they should certainly go. When the loss of a patient results in painful feelings, the doctor needs to talk to other staff members who were acquainted with this person, so that they can share their memories. Physicians who do not do so risk burnout (Holland, 2002).

When a physician approaches a family following a death, she may worry that the members will direct their anger at her. Yet when those who are widowed, in grief support groups, or chatting on websites are asked what doctors may say to help or what they should avoid saying, they respond as outlined in Table 1, as if they were addressing physicians.

The authors have discussed six stages of death:

1 Recognition
2 Process of Dying
3 Moment of Death
4 Departure of the Spirit
5 Care of the Body
6 Dealing with Grief

Doctors and other health professionals can help patients and their families at each stage, by considering tasks and completing the tasks suggested above. They can also help those involved cope emotionally and physically at each stage. As long as patients are still alive, physicians can help them approach death more peacefully.

A man's dying is more the survivors' affair than his own.
Thomas Mann (1875–1955), *The Magic Mountain*

I cannot say what loves have come and gone;
I only know that summer sang in me
A little while, that in me sings no more.
Edna St. Vincent Millay (1892–1950), *What Lips My Lips Have Kissed*

Between grief and nothing, I will take grief.
William Faulkner (1897–1962), *The Wild Palms*

Death may happen in a moment but grief takes time. And that time is both an ordeal and a blessing. An ordeal in the sense that grief is often of the most severe mental pains that we must suffer and a blessing in the sense that we don't have to do it all at once. (Colin Murray Parkes)
Agnes Whitaker, editor, *All in the End Is Harvest: An Anthology for Those Who Grieve*, 1984

TABLE 1

COMMUNICATE EFFECTIVELY WITH BEREAVED PATIENTS

Doctors can say or ask:	Because:
"I'm sorry," or "I'm sorry she/he's gone."	Acknowledges the loss.
"I can't imagine what you're going through."	No one can fully understand another's loss.
"What are you remembering about [the deceased] today?"	Bereaved patients are always remembering the deceased.
Depending on your relationship to the deceased you may say it was an honour to know the patient, whom you will miss	Bereaved patients worry that others, and even they, will forget the uniqueness of the deceased.
"How are you feeling since [the deceased's death]? How has [that death] affected you?"	Bereaved patients will appreciate the concern.

Doctors ought not to say or ask:	Because:
"Call me."	Passive effort puts the burden on the bereaved person. A sincere effort is to make a personal call to the bereaved patient.
"How are you?" (casually)	Ask only if you have time to listen. If not, don't ask.
"I know how you feel."	It seems presumptuous for anyone to claim to know how another person feels.
"It was probably for the best."	A bereaved person does not view it this way.
"Your loved one is happy now."	You have no way of knowing this and the patient may resent your presuming to know.

TABLE 1/continued

Doctors ought not to say or ask:	Because:
"It is God's will."	Those who are in mourning typically protest the death. Saying God wanted it this way may confuse the religious and offend the nonreligious.
"It was his time to go."	Bereaved patients have trouble seeing it this way. Those in mourning protest their loved one's departure and almost never think the time was 'right'.
"I'm sorry I brought it up."	Don't be sorry; bring it up.
"Let's change the subject."	Don't change the subject. Bereaved patients want to talk with you about their loss.
"You should work toward getting over this by now."	Bereaved people never 'get over' their loss but learn to live with it ... If grief is prolonged, it may be time for a referral for expert help.
"You're strong enough to deal with it."	Mourning is about the loss and not about the mourner's strength. A more appropriate response might be to say to the bereaved, "I hope you find the strength to bear your loss."

(Prigerson and Jacobs, 2001: 1373)

3

The Physician's Role in a Peaceful Death

There is a time in a patient's life when the pain ceases to be, when the mind slips off into a dreamless state, when the need for food becomes minimal, and the awareness of the environment all but disappears into darkness ... Watching a peaceful death of a human being reminds us of a falling star: one of a million lights in a vast sky that flares up for a brief moment only to disappear into the endless night forever.

Elisabeth Kübler-Ross, *On Death and Dying*, 1969

WHAT CONSTITUTES A PEACEFUL DEATH?

A peaceful death. These three words conjure up as many images and responses as there are people. In order to explore this area as fully as possible, the authors focus on the following questions:

- What constitutes a peaceful death?
- What constitutes a unpeaceful death?

And for those who have experienced the death of a loved one:

- Do you believe your loved one died a peaceful death?
- How was the physician involved in that death?

Some of the physicians in the authors' sample emphasized the patient's emotional and spiritual state when deciding whether a death was peaceful or not. Sally Knox, a surgeon specializing in breast cancer, considered a patient's death peaceful if "the patient has been able to tie up loose ends and is at peace in the midst of a storm." Alan Hamill, an AIDS physician, said a peaceful death was one in which the patient was "fully conscious and had a sense of completion in life and relationships. It is also a death in which spiritual needs have been met."

Others described a peaceful death as one that is painless, expected, with any final business completed. A woman physician said, "there is time to make arrangements and to react emotionally before death." Fran Blais, an infectious disease physician, described it as "one that is expected and prepared for, hopefully at home with significant others present: one that is as pain-free as possible; and one in which business matters have been taken care of early in the illness." Others in the authors' sample echoed that peaceful deaths occur when emotional support is present.

Some felt a peaceful death excludes certain types of death. An addictionologist put it this way: "No extreme medical measures were used. No death by violence or accidents. No sudden death." Medical staff sometimes use desperate or "heroic" efforts when the chance of recovery is almost non-existent; such measures include using ventilators, shocking a patient's heart, performing open heart massage and other invasive procedures such as central lines, and drawing blood multiple times.

Tina Bailey, a nurse practitioner and participant in our study, raised an interesting point regarding who should decide just how peaceful a death should be. She said, "I don't look at it as peaceful or not. I allow the patient to tell me what they want. If that means fighting, struggling, and being as alert as possible up to the last minute, then that's good. If, on the other hand, the patient is afraid of pain and wants to use medicines to the point of being sedated, then that's good. It's a personal choice. I try to respect the wishes of the patient and not project what is 'easier' for the professionals."

In *To Live until We Say Goodbye*, Elisabeth Kübler-Ross (1978) described those who struggle to the very end as the "fighters and rebels." She believes "it is important that we do not sedate these patients, that we allow them to ventilate and externalize their rage, their anger, and their need to try every possible medical and sometimes not 'socially acceptable' treatment." (Quoted in *Dying: A Book of Comfort*, Pat McNees, 1996: 25–6.) The authors agree that patients – not the medical staff – need to decide how much they want to struggle and hang on to life, how alert they want to be, and what heroic measures they wish taken on their behalf.

In her moving memoir *Heartsounds*, Martha Weinman Lear, wife of a physician who was dying from heart disease, wrote how he lived much longer than any of his doctors had thought possible, largely because he fought so hard to be given every chance (1980). Other patients, however, prefer to die quietly and painlessly. The authors believe physicians should make every effort to provide patients with adequate analgesics when they clearly want them.

Marilyn J. Field, study director for the Committee on Care at the End of Life at the Institute of Medicine (IOM), described the IOM committee's view of a good death "as one that was free from unavoidable pain and other distress; in general accord with patient and family wishes; and reasonably consistent with clinical, cultural, and ethical standards" (Berman, 1997: 502).

A qualitative study by P.A. Singer, D.K. Martin, and M. Kelner (1999), conducted in Toronto, addressed the question of what patients consider quality end-of-life care to include. The study involved 126 patients from three patients groups: dialysis patients, HIV patients, and the residents of a long term care facility. The domains, which the patients identified, were categorized into five main concerns:

Domain 1: Receiving adequate pain and symptom management (for vomiting, breathlessness, and diarrhea).
Domain 2: Avoiding inappropriate prolongation of dying. Patients didn't want to be kept alive after they could no longer enjoy their lives.
Domain 3: Achieving a sense of control. Patients wanted to make decisions, while they could, and to pass control to a chosen proxy when they could no longer make proper decisions.
Domain 4: Relieving the burden on loved ones. Patients were concerned with loved ones having to witness their death; providing physical care (which required spending money or arranging for babysitters for the children, etc.), and knowing what decisions to express in a living will regarding end-of-life care.
Domain 5: Strengthening relationships with family and friends. Most patients wanted to communicate about dying with their families, as they hoped to bring everyone closer.
(Singer et al., 1999: 164)

In a self-study program known as *UNIPAC*, the American Academy of Hospice and Palliative Medicine (AAHPM) describes a peaceful death as the completion of a series of four developmental tasks. The first task involves developing a renewed sense of personhood and meaning. People complete this task as they review their lives, tell their stories, develop a sense of worthiness, both past and present, and learn to accept the care of others.

The second developmental task involves bringing closure to personal and community relationships. As patients say good-bye to family members and friends, they express regret, gratitude, and affection. The authors of the *UNIPAC* study believe those who are dying should reconcile with long absent friends and relatives by asking for and granting forgiveness. Finally, those dying need to say good-bye to those they know in the community, at work, and in civic and religious circles, so that they can express regret, forgiveness, and appreciation.

The third developmental task allows patients to bring closure to their material affairs, arranging to transfer financial, legal, and social responsibilities to others. During the final task, the dying accept that life is over and surrender to death. They express the personal tragedy involved in their death and acknowledge the personal loss. The dying also need to withdraw from the world and accept their increased dependency on others as well as the seeming chaos that precedes death (Storey and Knight, 1998). The more of these tasks the terminally ill complete, the more peaceful death will be.

June Mui Hing Mak and Michael Clinton reviewed the medical literature and literature in general to discover the elements of a good death. The seven recurring themes they found are desiring personal comfort or relief from pain and suffering; awareness of dying; completing or accepting the timing of one's death; maintaining control, accepting death and retaining autonomy; maintaining optimism and keeping hope alive; readying and preparing for departure; and selecting where to die and living with this choice. Mak and Clinton conclude that these descriptions come from health professionals, such as nurses and hospice coordinators, because few, if any, studies have obtained data from patients. The concept of a good death in the medical literature is limited, because so little is known about dying patients' preferences (Mak and Clinton, 1999).

Susan Block has identified goals that many patients see as central to a good death. They include optimizing physical comfort, maintaining a sense of continuity with one's healthful self and continuing to feel valued and connected to others to the end of one's life; maintaining and enhancing personal relationships; finding the meaning of one's life on earth as well as that of impending death; and achieving a sense of control, while confronting and preparing for death (Block, 2001).

Block developed the following questions to help patients define a good death:

1 Regarding the meaning of illness
   • How have you made sense of why this is happening to you?
   • What do you think is ahead?
2 Regarding coping style
   • How have you coped with hard times in the past?
   • What have been the major challenges you have confronted in your life?
3 Regarding social support network
   • Who are the important people in your life now?
   • On whom do you depend and in whom do you confide about your illness?
   • How are the important people in your life coping with your illness?
4 About stressors
   • What are the biggest stressors you are dealing with now?
   • Do you have concerns about pain or other kinds of physical suffering?
   • Are you worried about you or your family's emotional coping?
5 Regarding spiritual resources
   • What role does faith or spirituality play in your life?
   • What role has it taken in facing difficult times in the past? Now?
6 Regarding psychiatric vulnerabilities
   • Have you experienced periods of significant depression, anxiety, drug or alcohol use, or other difficulties in coping?
   • What kinds of treatment have you had and which have you found helpful?
7 Regarding economic circumstances
   • How much of a concern are financial issues for you?
8 Patient-physician relationship
   • How do you want me, as your physician, to help you in this situation?
   • How can you and I, as your physician, best work together?
(Block, 2001: 2899)

Block also recommends clinicians ask the following questions:

• What are some of the ways you have found yourself growing or changing, or hoped that you could grow or change in this last phase of your life?

- What are some of the moments when you've felt most discouraged and downhearted as you've faced your illness?
- What are the biggest barriers you find to feeling secure and in reasonable control as you go through this experience with your illness?
- How would you like to say goodbye to the people who have been important to you?

(Block, 2001: 2902)

By asking appropriate questions, listening, and remaining open to the wishes and belief systems of their patients, doctors can help patients plan what they consider to be a good death. Doctors can also help patients to end their life on earth in ways that they choose. Physicians can help provide a safe passage from life to death in this way. In order to help patients plan and achieve a death of their choice, a team of social workers, clergy, nurses, family, friends, volunteers, and physicians need to assist in the planning and to provide the necessary resources.

WHAT CONSTITUTES AN "UNPEACEFUL" DEATH?

It is as natural to die as to be born.

Francis Bacon (1561–1626), *Of Death*

The most common answer that the physicians in the authors' sample provided was that an unpeaceful death is an unexpected death, a death for which no one is prepared. A family practitioner with AIDS answered, "a bad death is unexpected from a physician's and family's point of view. It is not possible to prepare the family for the experience." An infectious disease physician said this type of death is, "unexpected, unprepared for, unsupported, one in which loved ones had no time to plan."

A woman physician viewed unpeaceful death as "violent, sudden, or prolonged, either painful and/or associated with coma, or when other cognitive impairment precedes death." The authors agree that sudden, traumatic deaths, such as those that result from suicide, accidents, heart attacks, or homicides, are more difficult to grieve than expected deaths. These kinds of deaths, according to William J. Worden, leave survivors with a sense of unreality, feelings of guilt, the need to blame, complicated legal involvement by authorities, a sense of helplessness, and frequently unfinished business, such as regrets about things that were said or left unsaid (Worden, 1991).

Brady Allen, an AIDS physician believes that "these deaths may be painful, lonely, lingering, involve keeping someone artificially alive with a respirator, or complicated by fighting among family members and/or friends." Other physicians agreed that when family members argue or intervene at the last minute they cause a less peaceful death.

Some patients experience troubled death. Sally Knox, a cancer surgeon, notes that these patients "refuse to acknowledge what is happening, cannot discuss it with family members, and are not at peace with themselves." Alan Hamill, an AIDS physician, believed that these are people "who fought death just as they fought life."

Nurse practitioner Tina Bailey again stressed the importance of choice. She believes an unpeaceful death occurs when "the patient does not get what was wanted. Examples: A patient wanted to die at home and was sent to a nursing home. A patient who eventually died at home did not want CPR done when the ambulance came, but it was performed anyway. There was a patient whose family played religious songs while the patient was dying in spite of the fact that the patient had another belief system. Even as he was dying, the family also told the patient that his life had been sinful." The authors agree that when medical staff and professionals respect the choices of terminally ill patients, their deaths will be much more peaceful.

In their study the authors asked those who had a loved one die about the role a physician could play in order to bring about a more peaceful death. Some respondents stressed that more pain relief would have greatly helped their loved ones, while others acknowledged that pain was well managed. One relative, Johnny N., remarked: "I don't believe Mom died a peaceful death since she kept struggling to live. However, I don't believe she was in any pain, which her doctor made sure about."

Anthony W. said that while he wanted to know if his lover Gary was in pain when he died of AIDS, he couldn't tell. "If a doctor knows that a certain stage or process is painful for the patient, then I wish he would advise the caregiver as to what medications should be used and which ones are no longer needed. Gary had so many pills that it was difficult and sometimes impossible to get him to take them. Therefore, if he only seemed to be in pain, I would give pain medicines only." Answering a caregiver's concerns makes good sense.

According to the respondents, honouring the wishes of a dying person is the top priority. An 81-year-old woman, Elsie A., when discussing the death of her 87-year-old husband, said: "He died in his sleep after having a totally unnecessary prostate operation (in spite of his right to die letter)." A nurse practitioner, Tina Bailey, said about the death of a friend: "If the physician had contacted the list of family and friends already set up and had known how to access services better, my friend could have died at home. I was given two days notice to make arrangements, and then the patient was admitted to a nursing home against his will. He was very bitter. He had arranged everything, and there was a whole list of friends who would have assisted. But the physician decided to deal with family members who had not been involved until the last minute and did not care." Stories such as these dramatize the important role the physician can play to ensure that living wills and the wishes of the patients are respected whenever possible.

> You matter because you are you and until the last moment of your life. We will do what we can, not only to help you die peacefully, but to live until you die.
> Cicely Saunders (founder of the first modern hospice), 1967
> www.st-anns-hospice.org.uk

THE LAST DAYS OF LIVING

The last days of living are among the most important in a person's life. During the final hours a person, who was part of the known world and had an impact on others, moves to another dimension, which none of the living – except perhaps in near-death experiences – have experienced.

In this section the authors discuss ways that physicians and health care teams can provide comfort and support to patients and their families and friends at this difficult time. Medical staff can provide education about what to expect and how to handle emergencies, make certain patients are not in pain, and simply be there for their patients.

When Is Death Near?

Robert Twycross and Ivan Lichter wrote in the *Oxford Textbook of Palliative Medicine* (1998) that patients are likely to die within a matter of days when they are:

- Profoundly weak
- Essentially bed bound
- Drowsy for extended periods
- Disoriented with respect to time with a severely limited attention span
- Increasingly uninterested in food and fluid
- Increasingly unable to swallow medication.

The use of certain devices, such as ventilators and cardiac drugs, in ICUs and emergency departments (EDs) can make it harder for medical staff to know when a person is dying.

Kathy Faber-Langendoen and Paul N. Lanken, members of the ACP-ASIM End-Of-Life Care consensus panel, wrote that in the US up to 60 per cent of deaths occur in acute care hospitals: of these, 75 per cent occur after decisions to forgo treatment. When patients are in the ICU, the health care team may realize that death is a strong possibility. However, they must inform alert patients of reasonable treatment options and their possible outcomes. A patient's decision should override opposing opinions of family or physicians, no matter how well intended the opposing view may seem. Sadly, according to Faber-Langendoen and Lanken, 60 to 70 per cent of patients are unable to speak for themselves when others are considering limiting treatment. In addition, only 10 to 20 per cent of patients have living wills.

Prognostic models, such as that developed for the Study to Understand Prognoses and Preferences for Outcomes and Risk of Treatments (SUPPORT), exist. However, these models give probabilities of survival or death with a 95 per cent confidence interval, while some individual patients follow an inherently unpredictable course. In an ICU, death often follows withdrawal of specific interventions, such as dialysis, artificial feeding, and mechanical ventilation.

While everyone involved may know death is imminent, they may find themselves on a rocky road, facing many ethical and moral dilemmas as they decide whether to allow death (Faber-Langendoen and Lanken, 2000). The following story illustrates common dilemmas faced in the ICU, such as who decides to stop treatment and when they should begin to stop. Should patients have "everything done" that they request, even if treatment is futile?

Paul T., 55, had HIV, end-stage emphysema, and heart disease. Prior to entering the hospital with shortness of breath, Paul had signed a living will and discussed his desire to forgo any unnecessary medical interventions with his friends and his family, to whom he had given medical power of attorney. Two days after he was admitted, Paul developed a supraventricular tachycardia and severe respiratory distress. When JS entered his room, he asked her point blank, "Is this it?" She replied gently that it could be and asked him what type of medical intervention he wanted. At this point he changed his mind, telling her that he wanted to be transferred to the ICU and to have everything possible done for him, including intubation. Prior to intubating the patient, the pulmonologist asked Paul if this is what he wanted done. He stated that he did and so he was intubated. He then suffered a myocardial infarction.

His family members, who arrived later that night, were very upset that he had had been intubated. They felt that he would not have wanted the procedure; they could not believe that he had requested the current interventions. Eventually, the patient was extubated. Again, he expressed a desire to have everything done to prolong his life.

His family tried to persuade him to choose hospice care. In response, he remarked, "I have a dysfunctional family relationship." Despite the aggressive care that Paul wanted, he expired suddenly, several days after his extubation. The family members were very upset. They argued that, since his death had been imminent, he should have been in hospice, despite his wishes. This case illustrates how difficult it is to predict when death will occur, how a patient's wishes can alter the course of treatment, and that considerable distress may occur when the patient and family each demand a different course of action.

Nevertheless, patients and families need to know when death is imminent or a strong possibility. Twycross and Lichter explain about telling patients about impending death:

The patient sometimes appears to be unaware that the end is near. However, if he or she is already aware that the illness is terminal, there is seldom need to draw attention to the imminence of death. Some patients ask, "When will it be over?" and reassurance that it will not be long is often welcome. Others do not ask even when life no longer holds any pleasure or when the ravages of disease have exhausted them and they long for an end. For them, it is a comfort to be told that release is close at hand. Patients should be assured that they will be kept comfortable and will not suffer pain. They should be told that nothing will be done to prolong dying, that death will be peaceful, and that someone will be with them. This does much to alleviate fears that they may have about dying. Those patients who feel a need to fight to the end and who struggle to keep going may find it a relief to be told, "it is all right to let go now." In this way a difficult death may be transformed into a peaceful one (Twycross and Lichter, 1998: 977).

Families and friends also need to know that death is near. This allows them to say good-bye to the patient and have closure. Knowing also may allow them to feel that they are giving and caring for the patient a final time. Twycross and Lichter explain:

Even when it appears certain to health care professionals that the patient has very little time left, relatives may be unprepared for the death and are upset because they have not been warned. Opportunity for farewells may be missed, and this can cause considerable grief, leading to a more difficult bereavement. Therefore, care must be taken to ensure that all close relatives are informed that time is short. However, a patient who appears to have only a matter of hours to live may sometimes survive for many days. Because of the uncertainty of prognostication, relatively wide limits should be given when informing relatives about the imminence of death (Twycross and Lichter, 1998: 977).

As soon as the patient and his supporting friends and family know about the impending death, everyone involved can address the final care giving.

Normalizing the Dying Process

Although everyone dies, many people, including some new physicians, have never been with a person who died. The patient and family will benefit if the physician explains the dying process and what to expect, and finds out if those involved know how to handle any emergencies that may arise. The staff should also anticipate and have on hand necessary supplies (Emanuel, et al., 1999).

Twycross and Lichter explain the most important need of the dying patient: "What the patient needs is 'safe conduct' at a time when he or she must surrender autonomy and yield control to someone else. It is important to do nothing that infringes on a person's individuality or damages self-esteem" (Twycross and Lichter, 1998: 977.) Twycross and Lichter encourage medical professionals to create hope in a dying person by valuing him or her, maintaining meaningful relationships, and avoiding abandonment and isolation. They also discourage a "conspiracy of silence," as well as the use of words of abandonment, such as "there is nothing more that can be done." Instead, the medical team should set realistic goals and relieve pain and other symptoms. (Twycross and Lichter, 1998: 977)

Educating the Patient and Family about What to Expect When Death Is Near

The family will want to know how to tell that death has occurred. The excellent *Education for Physicians in End-of-Life Care* by Emanuel et al. (1999) explains ways to educate the family. The physician can explain that absence of heart beat, respirations, or a waxen pallor signal death. The body temperature also drops, pupils will become fixed, the jaw may open, and body fluids may trickle internally. Knowing these facts will help surviving family and friends stay calm when these physiological events occur.

As death approaches, the patient may lose her ability to close her eyes due to the loss of the retro-orbital fat pads. The eyes sink in and the eyelids can no longer cover the eyes. Unless this condition is explained, onlookers may find it very distressing to witness. During the last hours of life, patients also lose sphincter control and may be incontinent of urine and stool. This too can be quite distressing. A urinary catheter and rectal catheter may be helpful. In addition, the patient may lose his or her ability to swallow, as the reflexive clearing of the oropharynx declines. The resulting secretions can lead to gurgling, crackling, and rattling sounds. (Some call this the death rattle.) Knowing this could happen can minimize caregiver and patient distress (Emanuel et al., 1999).

Finally, the family needs to know that the patient may have a decreasing level of consciousness. Emanuel et al. discuss communication with the unconscious person:

While we do not know what unconscious patients can actually hear, experience suggests that at times their awareness may be greater than their ability to respond. Given a doctor's inability to assess a dying patient's comprehension and distress that talking 'over' the patient may cause, it is prudent to presume that the unconscious patient hears everything. Advise families and professional caregivers to talk to the patient as if he or she was conscious. (Emanuel et al., *Module 12*: 13)

These same authors suggest that when family members know what to say, they say such things as "I know that you are dying; please do so when you are ready." "I love you. I will miss you. I will never forget you. Please do what you need to do when you are ready." Or "Mommy and Daddy love you. We will miss you, but we will be OK" (Emanuel et al, *Module 12*: 13). Such expressions are comforting to most people. Emanuel et al. also advise that touch can heighten communication, so family members may show affection in ways familiar to the patient. It is quite acceptable for a family member to lie beside the patient to maintain intimacy. Families may feel constricted by rules, especially in a hospital setting, and so may need to know that it is acceptable to say good-bye in a way that is comfortable for them (Emanuel et al., 1999).

Being There

In *Sharing the Darkness*, Sheila Cassidy describes what it is that the dying person wants most of all from family and the medical care team.

> Slowly, I learn about the importance of Powerlessness. I experience it in my own life and I live with it in my work. The secret is not to be afraid of it – not to run away. The dying know we are not God. All they ask is that we do not desert them.
> Sheila Cassidy, *Sharing the Darkness: The Spirituality of Caring*, 1992

Sometimes helping patients is simple. Rachel Naomi Remen, who has worked for 25 years as a physician and medical counsellor, was giving a talk to a group of women physicians at a local meeting of the American Women's Medical Association. She made the point that when treating the dying, the doctor's humanity can be more important than the doctor's expertise. When doctors have nothing left to do medically, there are other things they can say or do that can be as important as a medical treatment. This can include listening, offering support and simply being available for the dying patient (Remen, 1997).

THE LAST HOURS: SYMPTOM RELIEF

Physicians should make symptom control their goal for the final hours of a patient's life, according to Jim Adam, a palliative medicine specialist in Scotland. Symptom control will help bring about a peaceful death.

During their last hours, patients will become increasingly weak, immobile, and drowsy, lose interest in food and drink, and swallow with difficulty. While everyone involved may anticipate this final stage, sometimes it comes on suddenly and unexpectedly. It is a time of high stress, anxiety, and emotion for the family, the patient, and the medical and nursing staff (Adam, 1997).

Geoffrey Mitchell, at a community-based hospice in a provincial city in Queensland, Australia, completed a chart audit study of general practitioner management of the symptoms of dying patients. He studied 7 males and 13 females, whose average age was 67.5. He found that the most common symptoms were constipation, confusion, vomiting, inability to swallow, coughing, reduced food intake, back pain, nausea, edema, generalized pain, pressure sores, rashes, and urinary tract infections (Mitchell, 1998).

In a similar vein, Raymond Voltz, a neurologist formerly at New York's Sloan Kettering Cancer Center, and Gian Borasio, a neurologist at the University of Munich, Germany, found the most common symptoms in terminal neurological disease are dyspnea, loss of ability to swallow, restlessness, delirium, drowsiness, epileptic seizures, myoclonus, pain, nausea, vomiting, and depression (Voltz and Borasio, 1997).

Mitchell discussed Australian guidelines for symptom control, emphasizing two assumptions:

- There is a pathological basis to most palliative care symptoms, meaning there is usually an underlying disease process.
- Treatments consistent with current palliative care literature are logical, when the pathophysiology of the symptom is considered. There is usually more than one acceptable way to treat a problem.

In other words, to treat the patient's symptoms, physicians must continue to examine the patient, determine the cause, and treat the problem. Doctors are needed at the bedside of dying patients.

Voltz, Borasio, and Adam and other experts offer the following suggestions for diagnosing and treating the most common symptoms of terminal patients. Medical treatment should follow a search for reversible causes of problems, such as pain, discomfort, mental anguish, and certain medical problems.

Dyspnea

Patients are naturally very distressed when they feel they are suffocating. According to Voltz and Borasio, this is a cruel and fearsome symptom and everything should be done to break the cycle of dyspnea-anxiety-dyspnea. They encourage reassuring patients that they will not choke to death because nursing measures, such as suctioning excess secretions in the mouth, will prevent this happening.

Jim Adam (1997) recommends treating the reversible causes of dyspnea, such as cardiac failure, and the anxiety that dyspnea can produce. He also encourages the use of general supportive methods, such as explaining what is happening, repositioning the patient, teaching breathing or relaxation exercises, and providing a fan or cool airflow. Opioids and benzodiazepines can also help when given initially at low doses.

Voltz and Borasio (1997) recommend that physicians relieve anxiety associated with intermittent dyspnea with a sublingually administered medication such as lorazepam, or with inhaled opiates such as morphine. If the dyspnea is severe, he recommends using midazolam by slow infusion, intravenously.

Twycross and Lichter write that many factors cause terminal dyspnea or breathlessness, which may not be relieved completely. However, in their experience, reducing the patient's respiratory rate with morphine to 15 to 20 breaths per minute relieves the patient's perception of being unable to breathe. Also, since anxiety is often a component of dyspnea, an anxiolytic such as diazepam can be beneficial (Twycross and Lichter, 1998).

If a patient has a cough with sticky secretions, nebulized saline can be used; however, this should be avoided if the patient has bronchospasm. Oxygen therapy can also be comforting to some patients, even in the absence of hypoxia. If the patient has constant dyspnea, opiates or inhaled morphine may also help. A more detailed account of treating dyspnea, which includes a discussion of terminal sedation, is found in Module 10 of *Education for Physicians on End-of-Life Care* (Emanuel et al., 1999, Storey and Knight, 1996).

Restlessness

Physicians need to diagnose this medical condition. Common causes include pain, a distended bladder or rectum, cerebral anoxia, inability to move, a reaction to benzodiazepines or other drugs, and nicotine withdrawal. The approach, again, is to identify and treat the cause, calm the patient and family, and, if indicated clinically, give benzodiazepines, such as diazepam (Voltz and Borasio, 1997). When nicotine withdrawal is the cause of restlessness, a nicotine replacement patch may also help.

For restlessness of unknown origin, Porter Storey and Carol Knight (1996) suggest lorazepam as needed or midazolam.

Delirium

Twenty-eight to 83 per cent of terminal patients develop delirium, depending on the population studied and the criteria used to define it. Delirium, a disturbance of consciousness, cognition, and perception, may be hyperactive with hallucinations and paranoid ideas; hypoactive with a decreased level of consciousness with somnolence; or mixed when the patient alternates between a hyperactive and hypoactive delirium (Casarett and Inouye, 2001).

Once again, the physician needs to find the underlying cause and treat it. Contributing causes of delirium include conditions such as hypercalcemia, infection, or brain metastases, psychosocial factors such as vision problems, pain, or unfamiliar surroundings, and medications commonly used for end-of-life care, such as opioids or corticosteroids. One intervention that can help reduce agitation due to strange surroundings is to encourage the family to remain with and calm the patient. David Casarett and Sharon Inouye (2001) offer other good information on diagnosis and management.

Hemorrhage

Family members and caretakers may understandably be horrified if their loved one begins to hemorrhage, especially if none of those involved have anticipated this happening. Medical staff can use green or dark coloured towels to lessen the frightening sight of blood on white sheets.

A member of the medical staff should take a compassionate approach, holding the patient's hand and staying with him, according to Twycross and Lichter. They also add that hemorrhage usually becomes fatal quickly. For instance, hemorrhage from a carotid artery in neck cancer results in death within minutes. Twycross and Lichter also discuss the use of midazolam and morphine to eliminate distress in this situation (Twycross and Lichter, 1998).

Dry Mouth

A member of the medical staff can prevent this very distressing condition by providing regular oral hygiene every two hours while the patient is awake, giving water by pipette or syringe every 30 to 60 minutes. Smoothing lips with Vaseline or moist air, treating candidiasis with nystatin, and giving the patient small portions of pineapple, ice cream, and crushed ice (Voltz, 1997) also help.

Loss of Ability to Swallow

When the patient can no longer swallow due to weakness and decreased neurological function, secretions build up in the oropharynx and create a disturbing noise. Relatives and patients – even when semiconscious – may be bothered by the sound. The patient may have dyspnea at this time, a condition that the physician should treat.

The doctor can begin by explaining what is happening to the family and to the patient, even if semiconscious. To control secretions, the physician can gently aspirate the patient's mouth and put the patient on her side. The doctor can use scopolamine in adults. The medical staff should avoid the term "death rattle," which is discomforting to families and caregivers (Emanuel et al., 1999).

Pain Control

Many doctors are afraid of pain control, fearing that they will kill the patient prematurely. Medical professionals apply the Rule of Double Effect, which Roman Catholic theologians developed in the Middle

Ages. They apply the principle to situations in which it is impossible to avoid all harmful actions. Consistent with the Rule of Double Effect (according to which the nature of the act must be good; the good effect and not the bad effect must be intended; the bad effect should not be the means to the good effect, and the good effect should outweigh the bad effect) administering high-dose opioids to treat terminally ill patients pain may be acceptable, even if it causes the patient's death. In fact, this rarely happens when the physician is following accepted dosing guidelines (Emanuel et al., 1999).

The rule does not allow medical professionals to participate in physician-assisted suicide, voluntary euthanasia, or, in certain instances, foregoing life-sustaining treatment. The rule does not condone terminally sedating a patient, as this invariably brings about death, or taking a patient off the ventilator, if the goal in doing this is to hasten or to cause death (Quill, 1997).

Twycross and Lichter believe that pain evaluation is important when patients are near death and comatose. Patients can feel pain even when unconscious. A common cause of pain shortly before death is withdrawal of oral pain medications because the patient can no longer swallow. For example, if a doctor withdraws oral opioids from a patient who has stopped swallowing, the patient will experience withdrawal restlessness unless the doctor replaces the opioids with analgesics, given as a suppository, sublingually, or subcutaneously.

Twycross and Lichter also note that dying patients, just before death, develop stiffness of their joints, so that any movement becomes painful. A member of the medical team can decrease this disturbing pain by gently and slowly handling and moving the joint; a short-acting strong opioid (e.g. dextromoramide) will also help (Twycross and Lichter, 1998).

The following books provide detailed guidelines in pain management for terminally ill patients:

Storey, P., and C.F. Knight. 2003. *UNIPAC Three: Assessment and Treatment of Pain in the Terminally Ill.* (Second Edition). Larchmont, NY: Mary Ann Liebert, publishers.

Doyle, D., G.W.C. Hanks, and N. MacDonald, eds. 1998. *Oxford Textbook of Palliative Medicine.* Second edition. Oxford: Oxford University Press.

Emanuel, L.L., C.F. von Gunten, and F.D. Ferris, eds. 1999. "Education for Physicians on End-of-Life Care." *American Medical Association.*

Ezekiel Emanuel, while at the department of clinical bioethics at the National Institute of Health, and Linda Emanuel, while at the Division of Ethical Standards at the American Medical Association, suggested that physicians assess seven domains regarding the patient's experience in order to determine possible interventions (Emanuel and Emanuel, 1998). These are their recommendations:

- To assess general pain, doctors should ask what symptoms are most bothersome and how much pain the patient has had in the prior week. They may find it helpful to ask the patient to rate pain intensity on a scale from one to ten. They may also ask if the patient feels over-medicated or whether the patient requires more pain medicine.
- Physicians also need to assess depression, which is very common. They may ask a patient how much of the time they have been feeling sad and blue in the last two weeks and what concerns are on their minds. They may also ask patients, when indicated, if they would like to talk to someone about the feelings brought up by the illness.

The patient may also be concerned with financial matters. Doctors might ask how much of a financial hardship this illness has caused the patient and the family. Has it cut heavily into the family's savings? In some situations, the hospital social worker may be able to make some recommendations. A related area is the care-giving needs of the patient. How much help does the patient need with bathing and eating? Will a personal aide be helpful? AC's mother, for example, required assistance each time she used her walker in order to help prevent a fall following hip surgery.

Physicians should assess how much family support and support from friends is available for the patient. Are there people living with or visiting the patient who can be companions or confidantes to the patient? If the patient requires assisted living, the medical team should help the patient find the best possible facility.

Part of the dying patient's experience involves spiritual beliefs. The physician may ask whether religion or spirituality has become more or less important to a patient since the current illness began. They may also ask if a patient belongs to a religious or spiritual community that helps her find meaning in life. If the patient is at all religious, his doctors might ask if he prays and what he prays for. No one should suggest that the beliefs of those who only believe in science and reason are inadequate.

Milestones are special events that can add great meaning to the patient's life. The doctor should find out if the patient hopes that a certain event will take place and if there is any way to help bring about this event. Sam L. wanted to visit his beloved beach vacation spot, where he had experienced some of his most memorable times, at least once more. With proper planning, which included prior exploration of local hospitals, physicians, and an ambulance service, Sam was able to do so.

Physicians can also assess whether any advance care planning has taken place. Has the patient created a living will that states preferences for medical care? Has the patient appointed a proxy who is aware of her wishes for end-of-life care? (Emanuel and Emanuel, 1998).

Physicians may not be able to control all the aspects of death that make it less peaceful; for example they can do little if a death is sudden or a patient faces death after living a tormented life. They can, however, play a major role in such matters as managing pain and adhering to the wishes of the patient.

GUIDELINES OFFERED BY PATIENTS
WHO HAVE BEEN NEAR DEATH

She enjoyed working with dying patients. There was something terribly real about many people as they got close to death.

M. Scott Peck, *A Bed by the Window:*
A Novel of Mystery and Redemption, 1990

Patients who had been near death spoke of their experiences to the authors, who then selected some of their comments for this book. The patients said:

- Tell me in person and have the physician be the one who tells me. This is very sensitive and personal information and I want to hear it face to face.
- I want my family to be there – if I think it will help me. Sometimes I'll prefer other supportive people, like friends or love partners. My family can let me know they will be there for me.
- Consider my state of mind. I want you to notice how I'm handling the information and how much I can handle all at once. Don't lie to me, but don't force me to accept more than I can handle right now.

- Be compassionate and gentle. The facts of the situation are harsh enough. If you seem too intellectual or cold, I will have a hard time believing you care what happens to me.
- Keep it simple but be complete. If you have to use any technical words, tell me what they mean. I'll usually want to know everything relevant but not necessarily on one visit. Ask me how much detail I want and remind me to ask questions.
- Explain the medical facts of the disease before giving me the prognosis. I want to know what is happening and why.
- Give me treatment options. I want to know what my choices are, the pros and cons, and what you recommend.
- Allow me time to make decisions. Set up another appointment so I can come back to talk some more. Usually I'll want to talk to my family or read up on the topic.
- Most important, give me hope. In most cases, I'll want to live as long as I can and to feel as well as is possible and maybe even beat the odds. Tell me the true statistics if I ask but point out my chances of doing well and what I can do to do as well as possible. Don't give up on me.

QUESTIONS FOR HEALTH CARE PROFESSIONALS

What have you witnessed to be a peaceful death?

SAMPLE ANSWER: A patient of mine died of AIDS. He had made peace with God and been reunited with his church. He was reunited with his family as well. He had adequate pain control.

YOUR ANSWER:

What are the characteristics of a peaceful death?

SAMPLE ANSWER: In my opinion, a death is peaceful when there is adequate pain control, the patient is aware of his dying, has made arrangements for his funeral, arranges to be with those he loves, and deals with religious and family issues.

YOUR ANSWER:

What do you consider an unpeaceful death?

SAMPLE ANSWER: I consider an unpeaceful death to occur when a person does not want to die, the death is painful, he or she has not dealt with religious or spiritual issues, or he or she is dying against his or her will by torture, violence, or war.

YOUR ANSWER:

Physicians can bring about a peaceful death if they understand and honour the wishes of their patients and provide symptom relief. Symptom control, as Mitchell explains, means making a diagnosis and developing a treatment plan that is based on current palliative care literature and is consistent with the pathophysiology of the symptom (Mitchell, 1998).

Physicians can't stop alleviating suffering just because their patients are dying. Patients need their doctors to remain at their bedside and to accurately assess and treat their symptoms, so that they can die a more peaceful death.

4

Treatment Options

There is so much we could do for our children and family members if our narrow mindedness and blinders did not constantly get in our way.
Elisabeth Kübler-Ross, *On Children and Death,* 1983

Today, traditional and complementary medical treatments are both available to the ill. Patients are so inundated with options, that they may be overwhelmed when deciding what to do. As the authors show in this chapter, patients make decisions based upon their values, goals for the future, and past experience with illness. Here are some responses from the authors' study:

One cancer patient, Mike A., decided against chemotherapy; he felt that the treatment would not prolong his life and would also make him ill, preventing him from having quality time with his family.

Johnny N., who had coronary artery disease, decided upon treatment. "I simply did not want to die without trying to get help," he said. "I realize that medication and surgery can prolong life."

A physician and an RN, each with HIV disease, decided upon drug treatment, which they felt was the best way to obtain more time with family and friends.

Patients want to live. However, they also desire quality of life. They must see their treatment as beneficial; the good must outweigh the bad. Susan D. decided upon treatment, even though it might grant her only one more year, because she had a new boyfriend, loved her children, and wanted to enjoy the final chapter of her life. She wanted and appreciated that extra year.

On the other hand, an HIV patient whom JS was treating decided against drug treatment. He had seen his friends undergo treatment and become very ill. Also, he disliked the way the medicines made him feel. He chose a shorter, but better life.

BLENDED TREATMENTS

People are criticizing me for my health foods and the way I'm caring for myself. Some laughed when I went through the Total Health Clinic. But what I learned there is helping me with the dying because it has improved the quality of the life I have left.

Ann Marie Johnson, *Meditations for the Terminally Ill and Their Families*, 1989

What is considered experimental today may be the standard of treatment in the future. In 1983, Elisabeth Kübler-Ross wrote about visualization as an alternative treatment. Now medical professionals consider visualization an acceptable way for patients to cope with pain (Kübler-Ross, 1983).

Norman Cousins received high doses of Vitamin C and used laughter to combat his illness. He described doing so in his book *The Anatomy of An Illness*, in which he describes his recovery (Cousins, 1979).

When he was battling cancer, Evan Handler was especially moved by reading *Getting Well Again* (1978) by Carl and Stephanie Simonton, and *Love, Medicine, and Miracles* (1986) by Bernie Siegel. The Simontons and Siegel observed that when individuals were "living out of sync" with their true selves, their illnesses were worse. They also believe that an illness can be a message that patients should heed. These writers encourage patients to recognize any commitments and beliefs that were causing them despair and loneliness and to break free of these bonds in order to get well again.

To help himself, Handler, while in the Memorial Sloan Kettering Cancer Center in New York City, employed a psychic, saw a family therapist, and met with a psychiatrist. Handler found that only after he faced his family's belief system, hidden resentments, and unspoken communication was he able to recognize and accept his family's compassion for him and to learn who he really was (Handler, 1996).

Physicians who remain open to their patients' desires for treatment, even complementary treatments, can better coordinate their care; they may even be able to guide them away from harmful or dishonest treatments. It is also important for physicians to be respectful of benign alternative care, as it may play an important role, by generating hope for their patients. Also, patients don't want their physicians to abandon them or label them noncompliant or ignorant if they experiment with methods outside mainstream scientific medicine. In most instances, as long as doctors are willing to respect the choices of their patients, those patients want to continue under their care.

A friend of JS, an RN with AIDS, stated that his CD4 count rose after he admitted to his family that he was gay, had a lover, and was HIV positive. He felt an emotional release following his confession, which he viewed as very healing. He felt that keeping secrets had used up energy; after he revealed his secrets that energy became available to him to fight his illness.

EXPERIMENTAL DRUG TRIALS

Patients may reach a point in treatment in which their progressive illness is expected to end in death. At that point no treatment approved by the Federal Drug Administration will alter the outcome.

A patient may then choose to enter a drug study, even if it offers only a very slight chance of survival. Patients may want something quite different from what physicians and nurses want for their patients (or for themselves). For instance, Slevin and colleagues (Slevin, 1990) found that patients with cancer required only a 10 per cent chance of symptom relief to accept chemotherapy. Their physicians and nurses, who were not facing death, required more than a 50 per cent chance. Apparently, directly facing death alters one's viewpoint.

Phase I, Phase II, Phase III, and Phase IV trials define drug studies in the US.

- Phase I trials are done to ascertain the safety and/or toxicity of the drug or agent. In these studies, a therapeutic response is not the goal or the expectation of the study (Sachs, 1998). Only a small group of people (20 to 80) participate.
- In Phase II clinical trials, the study drug or treatment is given to a larger study group (100 to 300 subjects). The Food and Drug Administration will allow a Phase II study only when it has reviewed Phase I data and concluded that the drug or treatment is safe for patients and that its clinical use may be beneficial against a particular disease or condition. Phase II clinical trials further evaluate effectiveness and safety of the drug or treatment.

- In a Phase III study, 1,000 to 3,000 patients test a drug. This large-scale testing provides a more thorough understanding of the drug's effectiveness, benefits, and the range of possible adverse reactions. Most Phase III studies, which typically last several years, are randomized and blinded trials. Seventy to 90 per cent of Phase III study drugs trials are completed and the drugs are presented to the FDA for approval. At this time, a pharmaceutical company can request FDA approval for marketing the drug.
- Phase IV studies have several objectives: to compare a drug with other drugs already in the market; to monitor a drug's long-term effectiveness and impact on the patient's quality of life; and to determine the cost-effectiveness of a drug therapy in comparison to that of traditional and new therapies (www.clinicaltrials.gov).

Patients want to be involved in a research study for several reasons. A new treatment offers a hope of survival. A patient may understand that even if he does not benefit from participating, the study may help others to live. Also, patients, especially those with no medical insurance, may appreciate the free medical care, testing, and drugs.

JS has participated as a researcher in many Phase III and IV trials for AIDS medicines. She routinely offers clinical trials to patients, including referrals to the National Institute of Health. Many of her patients, several of whom had CD4 counts of less than 10 and who were expected to die, are now alive and have CD4 counts of over 400.

Many illnesses have their own trials. (The appendix lists addresses for clinical trials for several major illnesses.) Clinical trials provide an option for dying patients who do not want to give up their good fight. However, patients need to realize that clinical trials do not guarantee survival, may cause pain and harm, and may make them feel worse.

COMFORT CARE

Greg Sachs, who practises Internal Medicine at the University of Chicago Medical Center, defines comfort care as care that improves the quality of life of dying patients by relieving their pain and other symptoms. Those offering comfort care are attending to the psychological and spiritual needs of patients and their families. Such care neither hastens nor prolongs death.

Sachs specifically distinguishes comfort care from hospice care. Hospice care refers specifically to a particular organizational structure for providing comfort care that, because of insurance and regulatory requirements in the US (e.g., the availability of a caregiver at home, less than a six-month life expectancy, and a low capitated fee), has specific characteristics. Sachs believes that patients can receive superb comfort care under the guidance of a physician, without being enrolled formally in a hospice (Sachs, 1998).

WITHDRAWAL OF LIFE-SUSTAINING TREATMENT

Patients (or if they are unable to do so, family and friends) may decide to stop life-sustaining treatments. Patients may decide that they have "had enough" and request no more treatment (Emanuel and Emanuel, 1998). A middle-aged man who had cor pulmonale came to the emergency department (ED) of the hospital where JS worked. He refused intubation, ventilation, and all medical care. He had been hospitalized over ten times. He just wanted to be kept comfortable and allowed to die. While JS felt uncomfortable watching a youthful man die, she followed his wishes.

A family that has decided that care is futile may ask to have care stopped, even though they are acting against the patient's wishes or best interests. A man in his sixties, who had been sick for several months, entered the hospital after an initial diagnosis in the ED of respiratory failure and renal failure. JS asked the man, in front of his family, whether he preferred life support or a DNR order. He chose the DNR order, but said he wanted to wait 24 hours before he signed it.

Within a half hour after JS left the patient, he had a respiratory arrest and was put on a ventilator, on which he remained for two weeks. The family then asked for the ventilator to be removed; the patient died within eight hours. The family members were comfortable with their decision, as they believed it reflected the patient's desires.

ADVANCE CARE PLANNING

There are currently three types of advance care directives in the US. Terms may vary in different countries or in different regions of a country.

- Living wills, in which patients choose statements to indicate whether they want to receive or not receive specific treatments.
- Proxy-designation – often called medical power-of-attorney – in which patients name a person or persons to make medical decisions on their behalf.
- Value histories, in which patients indicate their values and what gives their lives meaning (Emanuel and Emanuel, 1998).

In the US, persons have a constitutional right to have the above honoured (*Cruzan versus Director*, 1990). More than four-fifths of the US population, when polled, support advance directives. However, only about 20 to 25 per cent of patients have completed such a document (Emanuel and Emanuel, 1998).

Emanuel and Emanuel reported certain problems with living wills. The directives in living wills do not facilitate communication among patients, family members and proxies, so that proxies may not know the patient's values, goals of care, or specific preferences for treatment. Therefore, relying on proxies may not guarantee that the patient's wishes will be implemented and respected. Mark Garwin, a physician and attorney, notes that studies have shown that surrogate perceptions of patient resuscitation preference are often inaccurate, especially for those who do not want to be resuscitated (Garwin, 1998). Problems may also arise when living wills are not in the hospital record, the doctor does not know about the directives, or the directive is ignored.

Emanuel and Emanuel believe that advance care directives are not simply a document but a complex process involving many people over time. Advance care directives must be available, discussed with the patient, the family, and staff and used when needed.

HOSPICE

Hospice programs are designed to offer palliative care to dying patients and supportive care to their families in both home and facility-based settings. These programs attempt to address the physical, social, spiritual, and emotional needs of patients and their families during the last stages of illness and to assist families during bereavement (American Academy of Hospice and Palliative Medicine, 1998). In 1997, 3,000 hospices in the US alone treated 450,000 patients

(Emanuel and Emanuel, 1998). By 1999, US hospices provided services to 700,000 patients and their families. Now, more than half of Medicare recipients who die from cancer use hospices (Lynn, 2001).

Religious orders have, of course, provided institutional care for the dying for centuries. Cicely Saunders founded the first modern hospice – a freestanding outpatient facility – at St Christopher's Hospice in London in 1967. The staff members there use a multi-disciplinary approach; they take a scientific approach to pain control and pay attention to the social and emotional suffering of patients and their families. In Canada, the Palliative Care Unit at Montreal's Royal Victoria Hospital became a model for palliative/hospice care in all of Canada after it opened in 1974. In that year in the US the hospice now known as the Connecticut Hospice opened in that state in Branford.

Since St Christopher's opened, hospices have taken many forms, from palliative-care units in hospitals to home-care services provided in the patient's home. End-of-life care in the home is consistent with the wishes of most Americans. A 1996 Gallup survey reported that when asked for their preferences if they had less than six months to live, 88 per cent of Americans stated they would prefer to receive care and die in their homes (National Hospice Organization, 1996). Despite an increasing number of hospice programs in the US, only 20 per cent of the total number of patients eligible for the Medicare Hospice Benefit received hospice care, according to the American Academy of Hospice and Palliative Medicine (Schonwetter, 1999). However, as physicians become more involved and knowledgeable about palliative care, more patients are likely to receive hospice care.

Physicians may play several roles in providing hospice care. They may:

- Help patients and family members move from a cure-oriented treatment model to palliative care, if this is desired.
- Educate patients and their families about the diagnosis, expected course of illness, and available treatment options in a caring manner.
- Provide effective interventions, from managing pain to controlling other symptoms, in order to alleviate suffering.
- Collaborate with other members of the interdisciplinary team in order to help the patient.
- Help the patient and the family make treatment decisions that honour the patient's wishes.

- Offer emotional support and reassurance to the patient and the family.
(Storey and Knight, 1998)

Outcome measures are still a relatively new concept in documenting the effectiveness of hospices (Merriman, 1999). Nonetheless, a growing number of instruments are now available to measure pain control, other symptoms, and quality of life (Donaldson and Field, 1998). There are few evaluations of palliative care services (Greer, 1986, Mount and Scott, 1983) because many ethical and experimental design problems make this area of study difficult to measure (Calman and Hanks, 1998). However, guidelines for effectively conducting this type of research do exist (Max and Portonoy, 1998, Bruera, 1998, and Alexander, 1998). This is important because evidence-based research is just as necessary in this area of medicine as in any other. One study concluded that satisfaction with hospice care is associated more with quality of life than with the measurements of symptoms alone. Symptoms do become more important, though, during inpatients stays (Tierney, and Horton, 1998).

WRITING A WILL AND PLANNING FOR FINAL RITES

No matter what treatment or combination of treatments patients decide upon, physicians should suggest that patients write a will and plan their final rites. By writing a will, patients can determine what will happen to their assets. Even if they have only a small amount of money and no family, patients may want to bequeath their belongings to charity or to a special person. In a will, patients can also name who will care for aging parents, children, and pets. Patients may also indicate that they want to donate their body to a medical school or research, have an autopsy, or be an organ donor. This final planning can help patients feel in control at the end of their lives. Certainly, the existence of a will decreases the emotional and financial strain on survivors.

Deciding on final rites can also be emotionally liberating, as this forum allows patients and family to discuss openly the possibility of death and how everyone feels about it. Patients may want a special song or poem to be performed or to have a special person speak at their funeral. If patients make these plans before dying, there is less stress and uncertainty for all involved.

INFORMED CONSENT

Whatever treatment a patient decides upon, the concept of informed consent is important. Informed consent means that the patient has been told the diagnosis, the expected outcomes, and the risks and benefits of all treatment options under consideration, including those of non-treatment (Smith and Swisher, 1998).

Physicians can offer a variety of options to the terminal patient: experimental drug trials, comfort care, hospice, withdrawal of life-sustaining treatment, and complementary treatment as a supplement to traditional care.

Patients, of course, want quality and quantity of life and do not want discomfort. They will, then, use the treatments that appear to secure this and avoid the ones that do not. As one patient in the authors' study said, he was "allergic to pain."

Patients also need to make decisions about such matters as living wills and designating a proxy. As their lives draw to a close, patients do not judge treatments as standard versus alternative. Instead, they consider what works and what does not.

PART TWO

Interacting with Patients and Families

5

Talking with the Dying Patient

When you accept that you're going to die, you kid yourself a little less.
Priorities change; you look at life differently.

Allegra Taylor, *Acquainted with the Night:*
A Year on the Frontiers of Death, 1995

When speaking with dying patients, physicians should try to be as relaxed and as natural as possible. They are more likely to appear relaxed if they sit at eye level with their patients and maintain eye contact. Once physicians develop trust, dying patients will find it easier to talk about what they want. Doctors should encourage their patients to talk and will do so if they tell patients that they want to hear their thoughts and feelings at this difficult time. Doctors must not interrupt or correct their patients; instead, they should focus their attention on their patients and acknowledge what their patients are saying. Above all, doctors should listen, as listening is more important than talking in this situation.

Doctors should, of course, explain what they will be doing next. They may also share their feelings, admitting they feel sad or are at a loss for words. Also, they should not assume they understood exactly what the patient meant in a discussion but should ask if they are in doubt. When JS was a medical student in her psychiatry rotation, a depressed patient told a resident and JS that she would find a warm bath relaxing. JS asked her to explain what made baths relaxing for her. The woman answered that she would like to cut her wrists in order to see the blood ooze slowly into the water. The surprised resident told JS she was glad JS had asked that question, because she had assumed the woman just wished to relax a little.

Sogyal Rinpoche, the author of *The Tibetan Book of Living and Dying*, recommended two simple ways that people can release the compassion they feel inside toward a dying person. They can think of the dying person as someone just like them, with the same fears and the same desires for peace and serenity. This perspective can help them open their hearts even more than they already are. They can also put themselves in the dying person's place, imagining that they are facing death. They can ask, If I were this patient what would I need and want from my doctor?

Rinpoche also believes that health care providers should remember how much loss the person is experiencing: "Often we forget that the dying are losing their whole world: their house, their job, their relationships, their body and their mind – they're losing everything. All the losses we could possibly experience in life are joined together in one overwhelming loss when we die, so how could anyone dying not be sometimes sad, sometimes panicked, sometimes angry?" It is also important to reassure the dying that whatever they feel is normal.

Sometimes people cannot die at home, where they would feel most comfortable. In those situations the medical team should encourage friends and family to bring in plants, photographs, personal items, children, and, if possible, home-cooked meals.

The medical team needs to ask whether the patient does or does not want life support, to be an organ donor, or to have an autopsy done. Does the patient have a living will? Has he or she given anyone the medical power of attorney? What level of pain control does the patient want? Has the patient made funeral arrangements and made these wishes known to the family?

A study conducted by Harlan Krumholz and colleagues reported that only 25 per cent of 936 patients said they had discussed end-of-life care with a doctor. Surprisingly, such discussions did not improve the likelihood that the doctors correctly understood what the patients wanted. Krumholz et al. noted that congestive heart failure patients commonly change their minds about resuscitation when they get better. Over two months, 40 per cent of the patients who did not want resuscitation changed their minds. Doctors therefore need to continue to communicate with patients regarding these questions. Krumholz et al. stress the importance of timing. Doctors should not ask patients disturbing questions as soon as they are admitted to the hospital, but should ask them when discussing all the available treatments, so that patients do not assume they are going to die very soon (Krumholz et al., 1998).

Peter Ditto and colleagues interviewed 332 adults who were recruited from primary care practices in northeast Ohio and ranged in age from 67 to 97 years. They were asked about preferences for life-sustaining treatments in nine illness scenarios that they were shown and treatment versus no treatment and then interviewed one and two years later.

Ditto's results showed that preferences for life-sustaining treatments, though moderately stable over time, varied depending on the illness scenario and treatment. The patients' preferences for treatments were most stable for the most and least serious medical conditions and for decisions to refuse treatment. Health care providers should thus not assume preferences for life-sustaining treatments do not change over time (Ditto et al, 2003).

Physicians who are open with a dying patient, while respectful of how open that patient wishes to be, can help the terminally ill achieve a more peaceful death (Quill, 2000).

TELLING A PATIENT THAT HE OR SHE HAS A TERMINAL ILLNESS

The most essential thing in life is to establish an unafraid, heartfelt communication with others and it is never more important that with a dying person.
Sogyal Rinpoche, *The Tibetan Book of Living and Dying,* 1992

The authors asked the doctors who participated in their study how they would tell a patient that he or she had a terminal disease. They also asked the doctors how they would want to be given that information if they were terminally ill.

The doctors emphasized the need for gentleness when telling patients they have a terminal disease. David Donnell, an internist and AIDS physician, said he "asks them to sit in a setting other than an exam room and explains that he must give them some worrisome news about their medical condition." After telling them, he would then "discuss things that would make them feel better."

Another AIDS physician said he would tell his patients "directly and with compassion, allowing for questions and an emotional response." He would ask them to prepare a list of questions for their next visit.

An oncologist explained that she would tell the patient "honestly but with sensitivity to how a patient is receiving the information, how much information he or she wants, and with gentleness." The doctors would also try to present the facts in a hopeful manner.

Following are some of the comments that physicians and other health professionals offered. They said:

- I would try to objectively quantify the prognosis based on data. I would then explain that this data is only statistical and that many patients defy the odds.
- It is important to be honest but to err on the side of being too hopeful, especially at first.
- In a straightforward manner, I would explain the disease and the likely consequences.
- I would give them the stats. Then I tell them the rarities, the people who do not fall within the average. Then I talk with them about living with the disease and dying with the disease.
- I would develop a trusting relationship with the patient first.
- I would educate the patient first regarding the disease process before presenting the prognosis. After the initial shock wore off, I would want to see the patient again to answer their questions.

The authors also asked physicians when they would want to be told if they had a terminal disease. They answered:

- I would want to be told as soon as possible – regardless of stage.
- I would want to be told honestly – with my family present, and as early as possible.
- I would want to be told as soon as I became symptomatic. If I was told too early, it might generate hopelessness.

The physicians in the authors' sample did not seem to have a double standard as to how they would want to be told. They wanted to know as soon as possible, indeed at the earliest possible moment. Some emphasized that when dealing with patients, they might need to proceed in stages, depending on the patient's response. This makes sense, since physicians cannot assume that patients want information as quickly as they themselves do. Actually patients may not want the information all at once or too early. Still, physicians were aware that many patients do want the facts, as long as they are presented with hope.

Studies undertaken in the early 1990s showed that while most AIDS patients wanted to discuss end-of-life care with their physicians, only a small number actually did so (Teno et al., 1990, Haas et al., 1991). A more recent qualitative study, completed in 1997, which focused on barriers to communication during end-of-life care sampled 47 AIDS patients and 19 physicians in six focus groups. That study identified 29 barriers and facilitators to communication.

One barrier, which patients and physicians mentioned frequently, is discomfort about discussing death. A common barrier occurs when both patients and doctors wait for the other to bring up the issue. Some physicians fear that if they discuss death they may damage a patient's hope for recovery. Others were afraid that if they talked about end-of-life care, their patients would feel they were not going to be aggressive enough when treating them. The reluctance of physicians to discuss dying with their patients had, of course, been well documented before the 1997 study (Pfeifer, et al., 1994, Morrison et al., 1994).

Some patients feared discrimination if they disclosed their addiction history, homosexuality, or fears about being judged because of race or poor education. Others, who were still undecided about an end-of-care plan, feared setting a plan "in stone." Some of those who had made a living will felt that it was no longer necessary to discuss end-of-life care with their physicians. Some patients felt a need to protect physicians from discomfort.

Some patients and physicians even feared that discussing the end of life might be harmful or bring about death. Indeed, cultural factors may play a role in the belief that end-of-life discussions may harm the patient or cause death. A study involving Navajo subjects documented this belief among some Navajos (Carrese and Rhodes, 1995).

Following is a summary of the barriers to open communication, which the physician groups identified.

Doctors fear:

• Undermining a patient's hope
• Discussing AIDS with someone young
• Making their patients feel they are not aggressive enough in their treatment

Barriers also occur because doctors:

- Have too little time to discuss serious issues during appointments
- Believe their role is to make patients better, not feel worse
- Know that end-of-life discussions require considerable energy and preparation, especially since the many types of aggressive care make discussions very complicated (i.e., CPR, antibiotics, feeding tubes)
- Are aware that their cultural beliefs may differ considerably from those of patients and their families
- Are not ready for their patients to die
  (Curtis et al., 1997)

Proxies currently remain the primary way for medical staff to guide the medical care of patients who are not able to do so on their own (Morrison et al., 1998; Murphy et al., 1996). Of course, patients must be willing to discuss end-of-life care if they are to appoint proxies. A study conducted at a geriatrics and internal medicine outpatient clinic of a large New York teaching hospital asked 65 African-Americans, 65 Hispanics, and 67 non-Hispanic Whites about their attitudes toward proxies and noted which patients actually appointed a proxy to make decisions for them when they could no longer do so themselves. African-Americans and Whites were significantly more comfortable discussing end-of-life care than were Hispanics; 92 per cent of African-Americans and 88 per cent of Whites were at ease doing so, while only 49 per cent of Hispanics were.

In addition, significant differences were found among White, African-American, and Hispanic patients when it came to appointing a health care agent or proxy; 46 per cent of Whites and 31 per cent of African-Americans would do so while only 20 per cent of Hispanics would. It is possible that the Hispanics may have believed that a health care proxy is irrelevant because of their strong, involved families. They may also have preferred not to single out one family member as the primary decision maker.

The New York teaching hospital study concluded that if health care personnel and patients learn more about proxies, patients will use them more. Scheduling joint meetings with patients and their families may also help to promote discussions and decisions about end-of-life care.

Family physicians randomly selected in Franklin County, Ohio, reported that it is very important for doctors to communicate with dying patients and their families. Physicians tended to be more comfortable with their patients than with their patients' families. They had a particularly hard time communicating with large families and families in conflict. One of the most difficult subjects for them to discuss was breaking the bad news about a terminal diagnosis to patients and their families.

The authors recommend the following guidelines when telling patients that they have a terminal illness. Involved physicians will:

- Allot enough time for the talk
- Tell patients they want to talk to them about some serious matters, asking if the time is suitable. Sit down near and at eye level with patients and maintain eye contact when the discussion takes place
- Find out at the beginning of the discussion what the patient already knows
- Try to find out how much the patient wants to know at this time
- Invite the patient or family to pray, if appropriate and everyone is willing to do so after sharing the facts
- Tell the truth, without eliminating hope.

Robert Buckman, author of *How to Break Bad News: A Guide for Health Care Professionals* (1993), suggests physicians ask one of the following questions (among others), so that they can discover what the patient already knows:

- What have you made of the illness so far?
- What did previous doctors tell you about the illness/operation, etc?
- Did you think something serious was going on when ...?
  (Buckman, 1998: 149)

To find out what the patient wants to know, Buckman suggests physicians ask one of these questions (among others):

- Are you the kind of person who likes the full details of what's wrong – or would you prefer just to hear about the treatment plan?
- Do you like to know exactly what's going on or would you prefer me to give you the outline only?

- Would you like me to tell you the full details of your condition – or is there somebody else that you'd like me to talk with? (Buckman, 1998: 149).

Even after beginning to talk, doctors would do well to ask their patients if they are following what they are saying and if they understand. They should avoid technical terms, unless the patient knows them, and should explain the unavoidable ones.

Buckman reminds doctors to be sure to let the patient speak and not to start a new sentence or subject until the patient has stopped speaking. Doctors may encourage patients to speak by nodding, pausing, saying "Mmm Hmm," "Tell me more," or other facilitating words or sounds. He also encourages the physician to tolerate long silences as the patient often uses a silence to think or feel strongly. They will often then speak about what they thought or felt.

According to the authors, physicians may:

- Give information about the disease and the diagnostic tests, briefly and clearly, before discussing prognosis
- Ask patients to write down their questions and bring them to their next appointment
- Provide only as much information as the patient can handle
- Summarize briefly; then ask patients if they would like to discuss more about the illness or the diagnostic work up
- Offer hope
- Offer treatment options
- Provide statistics only when patients ask for them. If patients want them, doctors might explain that group data for a disease suggests that while they may live for only another few months, some patients have lived for several years (if this is true). This is appropriate since no one, even the physician, knows when someone is going to die.
- Remember that patients surprise everyone – even their physicians. (Shields, 1998, Torrecillas, 1997, Placek and Eberhardt, 1996)

HOW SHOULD A PATIENT LEARN ABOUT A TERMINAL ILLNESS?

I would like a doctor who is not only a physician, but also a bit of a metaphysician, too—someone who can treat body and soul.

Anatole Broyard, *Intoxicated by My Illness*, 1993

A doctor's most difficult duty is to inform patients that they have potentially life-threatening illnesses. Although physicians may search their hearts for a way to break the news as gently and compassionately as possible, they know that there is no way – no matter how much they plan or rehearse – to prepare for the reaction they may receive.

Depending on the situation and the individual patient, reactions will vary. For example, a patient who appears to be in good health and whose illness is discovered in a routine checkup is likely to react with intense denial, even disbelief. On the other hand, someone who has experienced severe pain over an extended period of time may actually welcome the diagnosis. However upset that patient may be by the news, he knows he can begin treatment now.

To prepare to write this chapter, the authors asked patients in their study just how they were told of their potentially terminal illnesses and what they would have liked done differently. Some of those patients did not know what they wanted. They admitted that they knew that there is no easy way for a doctor to break such bad news, even when patients want to learn what is happening to them. Denny W. who suffered from both an aneurysm and prostate cancer, admitted just that. He was very depressed after he was given the news about his illness. Still, he said he doubted that the news could have been broken to him in any other way: "I don't know how a doctor can tell you that you have cancer without the patient getting scared." While he was hopeful that his treatments would be successful, he wasn't really sure they would be. (He eventually died from the aneurysm.)

In Denny's ideal scenario, he wanted the team working on his case to hold off on any preliminary judgment until all the tests were complete. He told the authors that as soon as the results were available, the doctor should describe the case simply and discuss the treatment options as gently as possible. He felt satisfied that this took place in his case.

Jimmy H. felt the same. He felt very rushed for time after his physician told him that he had lung cancer, since his biggest concern was not the cancer but his wife's well being. He worried about what would happen to her after he died.

Anthony W., 38, was diagnosed with colon cancer. Even though he was told about his illness "immediately, with the facts and the prognosis," he admitted he lived in denial of his disease during the following four years of treatment and stabilization.

Many patients, when presented with the most devastating news of their lives, are treated with callousness and even indifference. Tim D., an AIDS patient, was told his diagnosis over the phone and in a very impersonal way. "I had no support with me at all once I hung up the phone," he said. "I was devastated. There was no one I could talk to. I wish the doctor had taken the time to meet with me privately and given me the news. Although the diagnosis was correct, I wish now the doctor would have told me to come in and retest. At least that way I'd have had someone near to support me."

Charlotte G., a diabetic suffering from kidney failure and heart disease, also felt slighted when first told of her diagnosis: "I was told bluntly that my kidneys were failing and nothing could be done. They told me I had one chance in a thousand of recovering from heart surgery – that the operation, if successful, would buy me some time, but that was about it. With both disclosures I went through denial, then anger. Doctors shouldn't play God. It would have helped me a lot more if my doctors had explained the symptoms of kidney failure in more detail, rather than telling me so matter-of-factly and bluntly.

"I want a knowledge of the disease, along with the symptoms and the probability of recovery. I want to be told about the treatment options I have available, both standard and alternative. If there is no chance for recovery, I'd like an honest timetable, so I can begin to get my affairs in order."

What is apparent from these comments is that patients:

- Usually react with anger and denial to any diagnosis of terminal illness
- May want physicians to be direct and straight to the point, or
- May prefer their doctors provide the news gradually
- Need their doctor to give them news directly – not via a letter, phone call, or a staff member.

When JS prepares to tell someone that he has a life-threatening illness, she does advance planning. She recalls what she knows about the patient, especially his strengths. She also tries to find a quiet time in the day to meet. She encourages the patient to bring a close friend or family member with him to the meeting.

If JS has known the patient for a while and has developed a friendly rapport, she does a reality check on her own feelings, because she knows that her own feelings of despair, guilt, or sadness could interfere with telling a patient bad news. She believes she must put the patient's needs first in these situations.

Occasionally, JS has asked a family member to interpret the news to the patient, although this approach has not always worked out well. When JS had to tell a Buddhist woman, whose language she could not speak, that she had a brain tumor, JS relied on the family to tell her. The family, because of their religious beliefs, would not tell the woman. As a result, the patient died without any knowledge of her illness or why she was growing weaker.

When JS meets with patients, she sits with them and offers them coffee or a drink, when possible. When talking to HIV patients, she first explains the concept of CD4 counts and viral loads and then provides the actual numbers. She discusses the concept of living with HIV as a chronic illness and how new treatments offer increased hope for long-term survival.

JS asks newly diagnosed patients how they feel about their diagnosis and if they feel suicidal. If so, JS directs those patients to an appropriate counselling facility. She also offers to help patients obtain HIV medicine, explaining that she has forms in her office to apply for medicine from state-funded HIV assistance programs.

When JS talks with the patients about treatment options, she asks them to think about the benefits and liabilities of each. She has patient information material on HIV disease that contains information about drugs and patient support systems. Because some patients feel more at ease talking with a nurse or other health care professionals than with a physician, she tells them that these professionals can also provide counselling and support at nearby agencies.

Many people react quite rationally to the news that they have a potentially fatal disease. Some do not, however. A patient whom JS treated went home, locked himself in a closet, and remained there for several hours, emerging only after his partner persuaded him to come out.

Many patients react to news of their illness with disbelief. One patient of JS denied he had AIDS, because he felt God could not have done that to him. He eventually agreed to take his medication, however.

A young woman, Lola J., who reacted with shame when diagnosed with HIV, isolated herself from her friends and family. JS and her staff encouraged her to call and ask questions or just talk. She also encouraged the use of outside support systems and counselling.

The most difficult patients whom JS has to deal with are those who refuse standard treatment. She remembers two cases in particular. One patient, who believed AIDS was a myth and antivirals a weapon intended to kill gays, left her office to find alternative treatments. He later died. The other patient, a nurse with leukemia, decided on alternative medicine treatments, despite doctors having warned her that agents such as Laetrile would not work. She also died.

A man in his late forties came to JS requesting treatment for a sinus infection, a diagnosis he had received weeks earlier. Because he had problems handling his saliva and could not swallow, JS thought he might have esophageal cancer. A barium swallow later that day confirmed her hunch. JS sat down and told the man and his wife her diagnosis. He was actually relieved to learn what he had. She referred him to a specialist for a biopsy and advised him to apply for Social Security Disability benefits as soon as possible, since he had no insurance. He did so, thereby avoiding financial hardship for his family.

The cases above reveal that patients may react to a diagnosis of possible terminal illness by hiding from reality, refusing to believe in the illness or intellectualizing, feeling overwhelming shame, refusing standard treatments, or even experiencing relief.

Physicians cannot, of course, just provide a diagnosis. They and their team should talk to dying patients and should provide financial aid information and referrals to specialists and support groups.

A therapist asked JS to help her friend, a young Texan who had just had a ruptured breast implant removed. During that surgery the plastic surgeon had found a malignant tumour. He told her about it, but failed to refer her for cancer treatment. After meeting JS, the woman, who was panicked about her diagnosis, became hysterical, throwing herself against the walls of the office. JS arranged for her to go to the M.D. Anderson Cancer Center in Houston. This referral eased her distress somewhat, partly because the Center offered financial assistance to eligible indigent residents of Texas. She received treatment there and is still alive today, although she did require a bone marrow transplant.

Finally, JS and her staff always attempt to follow up with their patients. They make sure patients actually met with the referred specialist and are suffering no side effects from the medication. JS also checks on their emotional state. The following chapters include methods that other physicians follow.

WHEN SHOULD A PHYSICIAN TELL A PATIENT
ABOUT A POTENTIALLY TERMINAL ILLNESS?

Numbers, science, and medicine all fail to answer a deceptively simple question: Why me?

Perry Tilleraas, *The Color of Light*, 1988.

What is the right time to tell a person that he or she has a life-threatening illness, given that timing is so important? Is the right time at the beginning of an illness or when symptoms occur? In their study, the authors asked spiritual leaders, friends, and doctors what they thought.

What Spiritual Leaders Say

In some instances and some circumstances, physicians should consult with the patient's pastor, priest, rabbi, or spiritual advisor after giving news of a fatal illness, with the patient's permission. Doing so may help doctors avoid some awkward or painful moments and will provide the patient with more of a sense of relief and peace. Most medical professionals tend to ignore or belittle the need to attend to a patient's particular spiritual preferences. This is unfortunate, even though most patients are deeply concerned with the spiritual when given the news of a terminal illness.

The views of the clergy who participated in the authors' study differed. (While some spoke according to their faith, others spoke from their individual points of view.) Still, nearly every spiritual leader to whom the authors talked agreed about several points. They felt that patients should be told the simple truth, without any twists of language or eloquence to cloud the issue. For example, Reverend Rodney de Martini, who works with the National AIDS Network in San Francisco, said, "I believe that a person should be told simply, clearly, and honestly what the illness is doing to them and what they can do to face the illness honestly and not lose hope or personal dignity."

Reverend Philip Johnson, a priest from Arlington, Texas, echoed this sentiment: "I am always more comfortable with the truth." Other members of the clergy expressed similar thoughts, saying doctors should "give the facts about the disease" and speak "with full knowledge of the truth" and "in the simplest way, but with the greatest amount of information." All emphasized that doctors should approach their patients in a simple, honest, and direct way. Above all, the religious leaders felt that physicians must not hedge, because patients prefer the truth to avoidance.

These members of the clergy also believed that patients need support, both while the doctor or a family member tells them they have a life-threatening illness and after they know. Paul Settle, a Presbyterian minister, said, "They should be told by their next of kin, usually with their physician and pastor present." Reverend Angela Ferguson felt that patients should be "told by their doctor, with support persons the patient chooses to have around them."

Thomas Harshman, a chaplain with the Disciples of Christ, said that while patients should be told directly and honestly, they should also be told about the healing process: "Knowing the medical possibilities does not preclude belief in healing – whether physical/spiritual healing out of the disease or physical/spiritual healing into death."

Knowing something about the spiritual beliefs of patients, even those who are not members of a religion, will provide a physician with some guidance when talking to patients about potentially terminal illnesses.

While physicians cannot live their patients' lives for them, they can provide some guidance, listen to their religious conflicts, and provide for pastoral care. Physicians will benefit by seeing the whole picture, not just the medical one.

Friends and Relatives Discuss Timing

> Often times of crisis are times of discovery, periods when we cannot maintain our old ways of doing things and enter into a steep learning curve. Sometimes it takes crisis to initiate growth.
> Rachel Naomi Remen, *Kitchen Table Wisdom, Stories that Heal,* 1996

The following deals with the reactions of relatives and friends to the news that someone they love is terminally ill. While all the aspects of working with a terminally ill patient are difficult, this area is one of the trickiest for medical professionals. First, those professionals must consider the emotional aspect. Relatives and friends may express the same denial and anger that the patient does. At times, it may even appear that they, not the patient, are the ones who were told they had the terminal illness.

When responding to the authors' study questionnaire, Juan M. wrote that his family members were very uncomfortable dealing with their father's illness. They told him he was very ill with liver disease but did not say anything about the advanced stage of his condition. The family then had to talk around or avoid mentioning the terminal nature of his illness when they were with him. In fact, some of Juan's relatives acted as though his father wasn't dying.

JS told a patient in his late twenties that he was HIV positive in front of his mother. She started yelling, "My son is very anxious. Don't ever tell him again that he's sick." Because she felt that he could not handle the facts of the situation, she wanted, even believed, that she could shield him from the truth.

Also the relatives and friends of the patient may want to know why they were not included when the patient was told or believe that the patient should have been told in a different way. This can be especially difficult when the patient did not want relatives there or when the patient is closer to his friends than to his immediate family. Nurse Tina Bailey wrote about a situation in which relatives arrived at the hospital to plan for terminal care that went against her friend's wishes. Both she and her friend were very upset. A patient of JS did not want his mother with him until he felt better, because they tended to argue. His mother did not understand his choice and felt left out.

Another source of emotional distress may occur when a family's belief system conflicts with that of the patient. This has been a major source of emotional distress for a patient of JS who is HIV positive.

JS once entered a room where a young gay man was surrounded by his parents' minister and church members. The group insisted on staying in the room while a doctor examined the patient. The group's spokesperson told her the patient was now "heterosexual," because he had found the Lord. JS told the group that she felt this form of coercion was not healthy. Needless to say, the family complained and she was removed from the case. Looking back, she realizes that although she disagreed with the family's behavior, she would have been wiser not to have expressed her views.

Other patients of JS, who did not denounce their sexual choices, found themselves alone and abandoned by their families. She encouraged them to use the AIDS Interfaith Care Teams and other support groups that could help them ease their loneliness.

Another patient who was gay and HIV positive permitted his family to be with him in the hospital but did not allow anyone to tell them he was gay or had AIDS. The parents suspected he did and often asked, but they were not told. They looked helpless, but nonetheless showed their son love and support.

Instead of offering their own views in such situations, physicians should remain neutral and nonjudgmental if they wish to help. They may offer counselling or refer the patient to pastoral counselling and care.

Family members may be in conflict with the doctor and each other about when a patient should be told he is ill and how much he should be told. One elderly patient of JS, for example, was terrified of cancer. Her children begged JS not to tell her she had lung cancer. JS explained that she had to tell the patient. When she did, the patient took it well and expressed concern about how hard it must be for JS to give such news to a patient.

Children, on the other hand, are governed by their parents' wishes as to what can be disclosed to them. Physicians may not be able to tell children their prognoses, if the parents are not comfortable with the children knowing what disease they have.

I'm not interested in compassion that is focused on my death. Real compassion supports my living and supports me when I express my true gay self.
                                        Perry Tilleraas, *The Color of Light*, 1988

What Physicians Say

Words are, of course, the most powerful drug used by mankind.
            Rudyard Kipling (1865–1936) in a 14 February 1923 speech

The physicians who answered the authors' questionnaire stated that they would tell terminally ill patients as soon as they were diagnosed about their condition and in person. They also stated that doctors should consider the state of mind of their patients. They wrote that they all took the time to explain the medical aspects of the disease, as well as the prognosis.

The doctors try to be gentle and compassionate and to present information in a hopeful way. They encourage their patients to have supportive people around them if they wished. These physicians try to describe the illness as simply as possible and in layman's terms. They attempt to be thorough and describe all possible treatment options. They said they allow patients and their families time to make decisions. They provide statistics to patients but often tell them that an individual is not a statistic and that no one fits a common mould. Finally, they tried to follow up with the patient at regular intervals.

Deciding when to tell a patient about a terminal condition is complex. However, the majority of the people with whom the authors talked to wanted to be told immediately upon diagnosis. They hoped for honesty and compassion. Also, talking to a patient and his or her family about a terminal illness often leads to conflict. Being aware of potential conflicts can help physicians to be sensitive to the dynamics of the moment and to be able to intervene if necessary.

6

Facing the End of Life

I fear pain, dependency, ugliness, and loss of control. Pity from others. Being tolerated. Doctors with tubes and shots and knives and drugs. I want my dignity! I don't want to crap my bed as my last act and be remembered wasted and helpless. I don't trust others to let me die in good season; I'm afraid they'll keep me alive as a semblance out of misguided love or duty. I am terrified to die – something in me is terrified of how I'll behave during the process. Will I wipe out all the good memories in the minds of those who knew me to the end?

David Feinstein and Peg Elliott Mayo, *Mortal Acts: Eighteen Empowering Rituals for Confronting Death*, 1993

FACING THE FEAR OF DEATH

Not everyone in the authors' sample was afraid of death. Alan Hamill, an AIDS physician who recently died, said, "I'd rather it not be messy, but I have little fear regarding death itself. I recently had a near-death experience. It was very calm, peaceful, and reassuring."

For most people, though, death is terrifying. Patients fear they may be extinguished into nothingness or that they will have to account to God for sins they have committed. The authors learned from those who participated in their study that what many people fear most is not the moment of death or death itself, but the process of dying a long, protracted death. They dread pain, misery, and discomfort, with no hope of escape except through death. They are also frightened that that they will be a burden to others; many would rather that death came quickly, with minimum pain and mess. Most of the people whom the authors questioned expressed fear about a drawn-out, painful death process. A patient with colon cancer said that what he feared most was "suffering great pain over long periods and losing awareness and being alone."

Second on the list of fears was the welfare of those whom the dying would leave behind. What would happen to them? How would they be taken care of, both emotionally and financially? A woman who was not ill told the authors that she would fear the effect it would have on her loved ones, as well as the process of dying. Jimmy H., who died from lung cancer, said he feared leaving his wife behind because he would no longer be able to protect her.

Other fears have to do with the effect of the illness on family and friends. The patient may fear becoming a burden, losing their role as head of the family or as a breadwinner, or being unable to perform sexually (Buckman, 1998).

Some of those interviewed were fearful, too, of being alone while dying, becoming a "vegetable," or losing loved ones. A woman who suffered from diabetes, renal failure, and heart disease said "the only thing that scares me about dying is prolonged pain or being kept alive like a vegetable." She explained that she believed "in the quality of life, not the quantity."

Some people feared losing their loved ones. Denny W., who died of an aneurysm, said, "I do not sense I have a real fear of dying. It does disturb me that I might miss out on a lot of things I could still enjoy doing, such as being with my family." Sheila K., who had AIDS, said she was afraid that she "would not get to see my kids have kids."

The authors thought that several of those questioned would say they feared what happened after death, but only two people said "fear of the unknown" scared them most about dying. One of them, Tim D., who was living with AIDS, was most afraid of what followed death, because "he wanted to go to heaven." The other, a woman physician, said she feared "not knowing what, if anything, comes next."

AC remembers thinking about death as a child and becoming very frightened. What he found most unbelievable was the idea of losing awareness – of not being able to think or to feel. As an adult, he turned this fear into awareness, awareness that life is both precious and limited. Although he does not dwell on this fear, he knows that his awareness will one day end.

Patients also fear the physical illnesses associated with a terminal illness. They may fear being unable to breathe, inability to move, or nausea (Buckman, 1998). Maria feared becoming paralyzed, so much that she preferred death to being unable to move.

Others fear losing their mind, feeling confused, or being unable to think clearly. Patients with this fear might prefer pain to being well medicated but "in a fog."

The treatment may also frighten patients. Will their hair fall out? Will their body be mutilated by the surgery? Will the pain be unbearable? Will they be able to accept their bodies after a colostomy? Linda C., a middle-aged woman with throat cancer, feared becoming unable to talk, knowing how close her tumor was to her voice box.

When asked what physicians could do to reduce their fears, patients in the authors' sample emphasized that they could provide compassion, emotional support, and pain control. They could also allow them time to be with their families. Their doctors could even help their families to prepare for the death. George E. said he wanted "honesty, compassion, help in being with my family and friends, and to be without pain." One physician said she wanted help with the practical issues, pain management, reduction of symptoms, and emotional support. Another woman said simply that she would like her doctor to "just be there for me."

Above all, patients want their physicians to listen to them. Doctors, then, can fruitfully spend more time with their patients, letting them talk about what is on their mind, listening carefully and giving time to say what they think. They can ask their patients if they have any concerns or if there is anything that will make them more comfortable and at ease. The patients are likely to respond, like the patients in the authors' sample, by expressing their fear of having to endure terrible pain and of dying alone without family. They are likely, too, to ask their doctors to be there for them and for their families when death comes.

Many terminal patients also feel guilt. Did they miss early signs of the disease, so that it is now too late to recover? Many feel such guilt because they do not know that in the case of cancer, biological predisposition, even in the absence of early signs and symptoms, is more powerful than lifestyle or health awareness in determining whether the disease can be cured (Tempero, 1997).

More than a third of dying patients may be depressed; more than half of those with advanced cancer feel sad and anxious. Clinical depression among terminal cancer and AIDS patients ranges from

20 per cent to 50 per cent of patients afflicted, depending on the study (see references in Shuster et al., 1999).

Suicide rates are also elevated among the terminally ill, in part because of depression and inadequate pain control (Emanuel and Emanuel, 1998, Portenoy et al., 1994, Breitbart et al., 1995, Allebeck et al., 1989). The prevalence of depression among terminally ill patients who want to die is eight times higher than in those who do not (Chochinov et al., 1995).

Very few of the terminally ill would consider requesting physician assisted suicide (PAS) or euthanasia, although a majority believes these options should be available to the public. In a study by Emanuel et al. (2000), half of the small number of patients who seriously considered these options changed their minds over a few months. Depressed patients were more likely to consider PAS or euthanasia, but they were also more likely to change their minds. Treating depression, a curable disorder, is therefore significant in doctors' work with the dying (Brietbart et al., 2000).

When patients reveal that they are depressed or are considering suicide, their doctors need to reassure them that they will do their best for them. Whenever possible, medical teams should honour patients' wishes, including those that involve where they want to die.

DECIDING WHERE TO DIE

I feel that the issue of where I am going to die is as important to me as when I am going to die.

Herbert and Kay Kramer, *Conversations at Midnight*, 1993

When the authors asked patients in their study where they would want to die, most responded that they wanted to die in their home. They felt they would be more comfortable and at peace in a familiar surrounding with their family, friends, and pets. Charlotte G, who had severe heart disease, wanted to be in her home so she could be sure no heroic measures would be taken.

Another study participant, Kelly E., who was in good health, explained: "I would prefer to die in my home. My home is where I am most comfortable and where my loved ones are comfortable being with me. My physician could help by prescribing medication, equipment, and nursing in my home."

Families preferred patients to die in a hospital. They did, however, feel that physicians should let patients and families know more about other options and how to access them. Family members believed patients should be in facilities close to their homes. They also felt that doctors should focus more on making their patients comfortable and less on giving second and third lines of treatment when death is near. A man whom the authors knew was upset when the staff at a Veterans Administration Hospital tried to force his brother to die at home. He felt that his brother wouldn't have access to adequate pain medication and ongoing medical support if he were at home.

Dying at home may not always be possible or wise. JS recently learned about a woman who died of AIDS in her home. Her only companion was her young daughter, who did not know whom to call for help after her mother died. This was a traumatic experience for the young girl, according to her psychologist who told this sad story. The situation might well have been avoided with good advanced planning.

To die well at home, a person needs a 24-hour caretaker, a clean and sanitary environment with utilities, nutritional support such as water and food, adequate pain control, and individuals to maintain the home and care for pets and children. Many people, particularly the homeless, the financially disadvantaged, and the elderly, simply do not have access to all this. If that is the case, dying in a hospital, hospice, the home of a friend, or a nursing home may be a more humane alternative.

Of course, everyone's situation is different and must be looked at individually. For example, a patient may want to die alone in a quiet room with no one present. If the patient's last wishes include being able to die in a way that reflects his culture, the medical team must respect his request.

Spiritual leaders in the authors' study believed that a person should not die alone; a dying person should have a circle of family, friends, and clergy close by. Reverend Rodney de Martini comments on this: "I think a person should face death in whatever place provides the most care, companionship, and love. I prefer home, but I also realize that a person's home could be isolating whereas a hospital or nursing home could provide an opportunity to be surrounded by one's new family (the caretakers) at the hour of greatest need. The person should be someone who is willing to be gentle, quiet, and loving with the dying person. This could be anyone from a stranger who is providing medical care to the person's spouse or partner."

Pastor Michael Pozar felt that company might inhibit dying: "My experience is that many people wait for everyone to leave the room before they die – perhaps some people feel that their loved ones are holding them back."

Where people choose to die is personal and meaningful. Physicians can help by allowing patients, if possible, to die where they believe that they would be most comfortable.

Other studies agree with what the authors found in their study: that Americans want to live their last days at home. However, the same studies have shown that most Americans die in hospitals and in nursing homes (Townsend, 1990, McCormick, 1991).

Project SUPPORT, a study that examined the terminal care of patients in five teaching hospitals, found that the local health-care systems, rather than patients' wishes, tend to determine where people die. The greater the bias for hospital-oriented care during end-of-life in a region, the more likely the patient is to die in a hospital. Likewise, when there is more money available for hospice or nursing home facilities in a region, more people use the services. Patient preferences had little effect on where the patient died (Pritchard, 1998). It appears that for patients to die where they choose requires strong patient advocacy.

How people die frequently causes more fear than death itself. They may fear enduring pain and physical symptoms, abandoning loved ones, dying alone, feeling confused, or encountering the unknown. Medical professionals should reassure patients that they will address all their concerns, as well as they can. Since more than a third of dying patients may be depressed and suicide rates are elevated, doctors should also treat depression. While most patients prefer to die at home, their families worry that if they do so, they will not have access to pain medications and ongoing medical support. If a person is likely to die alone, for lack of family and friends, a hospital or a nursing home may provide companionship and support. Certainly, no one should have to die alone and in pain. Whenever feasible, the patient should decide where to die.

QUESTIONS FOR HEALTH CARE PROFESSIONALS

Where would you want to be when you died?

SAMPLE ANSWER: I would want to die at home as long as my medical needs for pain control were met.

YOUR ANSWER:

Who would you want to be with you?

SAMPLE ANSWER: My spouse and my pets.

YOUR ANSWER:

Do you routinely ask your terminally ill patients where they want to die and whom do they want with them? Why or why not?

SAMPLE ANSWER: Yes, by doing so, I can help them make these arrangements.

YOUR ANSWER:

7

Death in the Emergency Department

It is the recognition that the *real* event taking place at the end of our life is our death, not the attempts to prevent it.

Sherwin Nuland, *How We Die*, 1994

When someone dies in the Emergency Department (ED), the medical team faces a special set of problems when they notify family members and then deal with their grief. The impersonal nature of the ED, the lack of a relationship between the physician and the patient and his/her family, and the suddenness of the death combine to make talking about the death to the family especially difficult (Rutkowski, 2002).

An ED staff tends to be very busy handling everything from sore throats to twisted knees and everyone from accident victims to attempted suicides. Though not intentional, ED staff members may be hurried or abrupt when they first encounter the patient's family.

Many ED patients are young. Their deaths, whether caused by car crash, suicide, or some other type of accident, may often be alcohol or drug related. ED physicians, in addition to responding to the family's grief, must also deal with the denial of family members when they learn that alcohol or drugs played a part in the death.

ED physicians and nurses must handle a family's grief, whether they have been trained to do so or not. Following are some suggestions on how to contact the family (Edlich and Kübler-Ross, 1992, Walters, 1991).

- Only an experienced physician or nurse should phone the family, if that is the only way the hospital can inform a family of an accident or death. Robert Malacrida interviewed the families of 390 patients who died in the ICU at San Giouanni Hospital in

Bellizona, Switzerland. Regardless of the cause of death, those who received the news by telephone reported more dissatisfaction than others. Families seem to prefer to be told face to face about a death (Malacrida, 1998).

- The caller must clearly and briefly state his or her name, the name of the hospital, the name of the injured or deceased, and what occurred. The full severity of the injuries should be discussed in person.
- It is preferable for a police officer to make the initial contact in person when circumstances warrant it.
- The caller or police officer should advise relatives not to drive to the hospital alone, as they are likely to be emotionally upset and to drive carelessly.

JS remembers that the father of a young couple had a major heart attack. Despite bad weather, the couple decided to drive from Deming, New Mexico, to Albuquerque, New Mexico, a considerable drive, in order to be with him. Their car slid off an icy road during the drive and they were both killed.

PREPARING TO TALK WITH THE FAMILY

One of hardest things a physician has to do is to talk to the family of someone who died in the ED. The physician must switch gears quickly, which is difficult. One moment the doctor is frantically trying to revive a patient with major trauma; the next moment she is facing an emotionally distraught family.

Before meeting the family, the doctor should take a few moments, breathe deeply, and assess the situation. Feelings of frustration, limitation, and inadequacy are normal considering what is happening. It may be useful to make a few notes that summarize the trauma and explain why the patient did not respond to treatment. The notes will help to keep the discussion on track and allow the doctor to be less flustered when meeting the family.

When possible, doctors ought to find out the names of the family members before meeting them as well as whatever they can about their reactions to what just happened. Doing so will help make the initial contact less impersonal, thereby benefiting all involved. If necessary, doctors should change any clothing or hospital uniform that has traces of blood on it.

TALKING WITH THE FAMILY

Doctors will find that it helps to talk to the family in an appropriate setting. The head nurse can help arrange for the family to be taken to a private room when they arrive. The room should have a telephone, appropriate décor and furniture, and enough chairs for everyone to sit. If possible, coffee, tea and/or fruit drinks should be available. The hospital staff should treat all family, friends, or partners with courtesy, remembering this may be the worst day of their lives.

AC consulted at a hospital ICU, where he dealt with those who had attempted suicide. Whenever the family was present at the time of the evaluation, he met with them in a private, comfortable room to gather information and to orient the family as to available options.

When speaking with a family, a doctor might bring along a couple of members of the ED staff. He should introduce himself and the ED staff to the family. Everyone should sit down, even if they can only stay a few minutes. If the doctor seems hurried, he will give the family the impression that speaking to them isn't important, that they're an intrusion into his busy schedule.

Before the doctor shares what happened in the emergency department, the doctor should ask the family for their view of what went on. The doctor and medical team may be able to clarify some issues for them at this time. More important, though, they should allow the family members to feel as if they have been heard.

When the family is finished speaking, the doctor can begin to give an assessment of what happened, in clear and simple terms. She can explain the actions she took on the patient's behalf and how the patient responded. If available, the ED nurse may be able to shed light on what took place before the doctor was involved in the procedure.

Everyone involved should make eye contact with the family while speaking and respond in as direct and honest a way as possible when responding to any questions. The family, which may be quite animated at this stage, should be allowed to express their feelings and emotions. When they have finished with their questions, the team can respectfully end the session.

REACTING TO THE FAMILY'S GRIEF

Grief usually begins immediately following a death. When Sam L., a young AIDS patient arrived at the ED, he was having seizures. Although he had lymphoma in his brain, it was believed to be in remission. While he was still alive, JS talked to the family, explaining the young man's progress. After he died later that night from a herniation, JS took time to listen to the family's sorrow and anger.

Chaplain Tom Harshman of Fort Worth, a clergyman who took part in the authors' study, advises physicians to "realize that anger directed at the physician is part of the grieving process, so there is no need to get defensive. It is best to be responsive to what they are expressing." Families often do lash out in anger. A well-respected colleague of JS made a valiant effort to save a man who came to the hospital after he had been hit by a large truck that lost control on an icy road. The wife, who arrived after the man died, said angrily, "Why did you call us to the emergency department? We should have been sent directly to the morgue!"

If on arrival at the ED the patient is alive but requires immediate care, allow the family to see him or her, as it may be their last chance to do so. Some hospitals allow the family to remain throughout the resuscitation process. Doctors must, of course, follow their hospital's procedures.

If the patient dies, the staff should allow family members time alone with their loved one. Before bringing the family in to see the patient, one of the medical team ought to remove any blood from the area and any tubes from the body. One of the team members should also explain to the family that they may say goodbye to their loved one in their own way, by kissing, touching, or holding them. Some people, because of their immediate shock and grief, may prefer just to be left alone and to be silent.

ENCOURAGING CRYING

The family will appreciate a doctor's genuine support, honesty, and understanding. The most important thing a physician can do is to allow family members their emotions and tears. The touch of a hand or a reassuring grasp of a shoulder will go a long way. Family members need to know they're not alone.

Also, there's no need for doctors to remain stoic when they are genuinely sad. A doctor may find it helpful to remember that she was the one who fought to save the patient or he was the one who had to tell the family the patient didn't make it.

This is not the time for platitudes or false sympathy, both of which may appear condescending, or talking for the sake of talking. There may be no need to say much. (See the section on Dealing with Grief, Chapter 2, page 29 for more suggestions on talking with the family.)

COORDINATING THE CARE OF THE BODY

The medical team must care respectfully for the body after death to avoid hurting or slighting the family. Once everyone has taken the time needed to view the body, the doctor should make himself available for any further questions. He should not, however, give medication to anyone in the family who appears to be very upset unless he knows that person's medical history well.

After a death the ED physician or staff notifies the coroner's office and the patient's personal physician or family physician, having obtained the number from the family. A social worker, if available, can help the family by providing useful phone numbers, making them aware of counselling services that specialize in working with grieving families, and information regarding Social Security, insurance, or other available benefits.

A member of the medical team should discuss the need for an autopsy, especially in the case of major trauma. Since the word "autopsy" often carries a negative connotation, explain that an autopsy is "an examination after death done by a specialist" and that it can help determine the exact cause of death.

Since the family has just begun to adjust to a serious loss, the doctor or nurse should not use any pressure when discussing the possibility of organ donation. If the driver's licence of a patient does not state that he or she wishes to be an organ donor, someone can explain to the family that they can offer the organs on behalf of their loved one. This lets the family know that even in their grief, they still have the opportunity to give to someone else. Many relatives are more than willing to do so, unless there are religious or cultural restrictions.

Doctors should arrange to speak to the family in a private room, sitting down even if only for a few minutes. They should be accompanied, if possible, by other members of the ED staff. The doctor should begin by asking the family for their view about what happened, and, after listening to their responses, should explain clearly what was done for the patient and how the patient responded. As the meeting continues, the medical team ought to allow the family to express their feelings freely and should accept that anger is a common response to major loss. Physicians can accept, too, that their own frustration and sense of inadequacy are common responses to losing a patient. The team will then respectfully care for the body.

8

Death and Children

A man, though he dies before his time, shall be at rest, for an honoured old age does not depend upon the length of time, nor is it measured by the number of one's years ... Being perfected in a little while, he fulfilled long years, for his soul pleased the Lord.

Wisdom of Solomon, 4:7–8, 13–14

THE DEATH OF A CHILD

The death of child, adolescent, or infant is extremely painful and emotionally wrenching for families. Most parents will tell you the death of a child, whether just a toddler or an adolescent, is even harder to bear than the death of a spouse. The pain cuts much deeper because parents bring their children into the world, so the death means that they have lost both the child and a part of themselves. A childhood friend of JS died of renal failure when she was a teenager. Her father, who had adored his daughter, was devastated. He literally drank himself to death.

Marcia Friedman, author of *The Story of Josh*, describes how the death of her college-age son Josh affected her and her family: "A catastrophic illness of this sort, which bursts without warning upon a family, traumatizes all the members of the family. As in a physical explosion, the epicentre receives the greatest damage, but the shock waves extend outward – cracking, damaging, threatening. The extended family, friends, acquaintances and the medical personnel involved are all affected to various degrees" (Friedman, 1974: 4).

How do physicians tell parents that their beloved child has a life-threatening illness or is dead? If possible they should inform the parents together, promptly and personally and in a private and comfortable place. They should sit down with them and let them know that they want to spend time with them. When JS was a senior medical student, a physician's daughter collapsed in a gym. The ED physician emerged periodically to inform the physician parent about his daughter's condition. When it was clear she had no brain activity, the child's family decided to stop the code. The family members were ready, because the ED physician had kept them involved.

Though not a pediatrician, JS often has to tell parents that an adult child is dying or has died. She usually sits down with the parents in a private room and explains to them what is happening in the ICU. She finds it helpful to provide medical information, to explain the illness, and to be honest about the prognosis. If the patient has died, she attempts to explain what caused the death.

Families want to believe their doctor cares. Doctors may show that they do by spending time with the family, listening and sharing their own feelings. They may tell the parents what the child meant to them as a doctor and what they learned from the child. Doctors may, if it seems appropriate, hug the parent or touch his arm. They will, of course, not do anything that seems fake or phony.

When JS was a resident, a 17-year-old died of complications from a sinus infection that had not been diagnosed in a timely manner. The infectious disease physician was so upset by this teenager's death that he cried while sitting with the family. The parents were touched and moved by his genuine expression of emotion. Doctors do cry.

Physicians can also inform parents about support groups and counselling for those who have lost children and encourage them to call with questions.

Physicians may also want to meet with the family after the autopsy results are available, to go over them. If a child died of a genetic disorder, such as sickle-cell anemia, the parents may be concerned for their other children. Physicians may be able to explain the realities or offer genetic counselling.

When it comes to the death of a child, there are no reasonable explanations as far as the family is concerned. While doctors are doing their best to console and comfort parents and family, they are probably feeling a wide range of emotions themselves: sadness, anger, frustration, inadequacy, and sorrow. Doctors find coping especially difficult when parents and family are angry with them – even if they did nothing wrong, even if they exhausted the treatment options. Many doctors will find it hard not to answer back or defend themselves when they are also feeling hurt. At that moment it may help doctors to remember that the anger of the anguished parents and family is right at the surface; if the doctor is the only one with them, they may receive the brunt of the anger. In subsequent stages of the grieving process, the parents and family unfortunately often direct the anger toward each other, believing that if a different decision had been made in the past, the child's life would have been saved.

It's important as well that doctors remember to care for their own needs. If they have a colleague with whom they feel comfortable, they might open up to them about what they are feeling. If they believe they may need outside help, they ought to avail themselves of it. Some physicians dealing with death do not seek professional help, or even counsel from a trusted friend or colleague. They believe toughing it out is the "professional" thing to do. Many physicians who don't seek help wind up abusing alcohol or other drugs to numb their feelings. Most doctors know colleagues who have been suspended or lost their licences because of addiction. When doctors feel that they are damming up their emotions, they would be wise to seek help as soon as they can. Both the doctors and their patients will benefit. (See chapters 11 to 19 for more information on how doctors can take care of themselves.)

HOW A CHILD DEALS WITH DEATH

Out of the mouths of babes and sucklings has thou ordained strength.
Psalm 8:2

When Someone Close to a Child Dies

Just as adult family members and doctors need help coping with death, so do children who have lost a loved one. If death is unfathomable to an adult, it is even more so to a child. They may not understand the death of someone else or the possibility of their own death in the same way that adults do.

JS remembers that death frightened her when she was a child. She worried that she would die, especially when she went to sleep. One night she had to sleep in the bed in which her uncle had died just a few days earlier. She was afraid that because she was in that bed, death would take her as well. She was amazed when she woke up in the morning and realized she had lived through the night.

Children often know what is going on when someone is dying. One day JS was telling an adult woman that her mother had lung cancer. She had told JS that her young daughter, who was about ten, could stay in the room. JS was trying to be hopeful. But the young girl cut through the sugarcoating asking, "Is Grandma going to die?"

Children can sense when their loved ones are upset and when something is wrong. They have a right to honest answers to their questions, assuming their parents have given their consent to members of the medical team telling them the truth. Without the truth they will guess at what the doctors are not telling them, imaginings that may be worse than reality.

Most children go through three stages of bereavement. The first stage is the awareness of the death. During this stage they will ask many questions. While the questions may seem very simple, someone – usually a family member – must answer them promptly and honestly. If their parents have died, children may ask the following:

- Why did Mommy/Daddy die?
- Where are they now?
- What made them die?
- Will they come back?
- Can it happen to me? Was it my fault?
- Who will take care of me now?

If the child wants to view the body, doing so can be helpful. However, a child or adolescent should never be forced to view the body. Even an adult who is grieving a spouse who has just died should consider the needs of the child who has lost a parent first. Sometimes this does not happen, unfortunately. AC counselled a young mother whose close relative had died. She took her five-year-old son with her to the funeral in another city, just so he would "make her laugh" and help her with her grief. When asked if she was concerned about her child, she replied that she wasn't because he could handle himself and liked to help his mother. She had forgotten that this little boy was not an adult and he would need help in understanding death.

The second stage of bereavement is mourning. Children should be supported during this stage, when they express some of their sadness. The living parent should share his or her sadness and memories of the deceased openly and encourage discussion about the deceased parent. If a parent is unsure how to act or what to say, he should share this with the child. Children may want to draw pictures to express their feelings or make cards for the deceased person. They should certainly be allowed to cry.

Parents should remember that children may react to loss more intensely than adults. The loss of a favourite toy, a pet, or a friend, or a move from a house or neighbourhood may sadden a child deeply. A child will feel profoundly the loss of someone as important as a parent or close relative.

J. W. Worden (2002), a leading expert on grief, believes that children mourn in different ways depending upon their developmental stage. While children between the ages of two and five are distressed by a loss, they are even more likely to blame themselves for the death because of their imagined "badness." As a result, they are particularly vulnerable to failure to mourn adequately, becoming depressed and sometimes experiencing difficulties forming intimate relationships when they are adults. Children ages seven and older mourn like adults.

Finally, mourning in childhood is frequently incomplete and can be triggered anew during significant life events, as the child grows up. The tasks of grieving discussed in chapter 2 apply to children as well; they need, however, to be adapted depending upon the child's developmental stage.

The third stage of bereavement involves the resumption of normal activities. During this stage children need a consistent adult figure who attends to their daily needs. Children will probably reassess the loss of their loved one at each developmental stage. It is important to make minimal changes in the child's environment and daily activities (Mahon, 1994, Trimm, 1995) during all stages of mourning.

The stages of recognition, mourning, and resuming normal activities can overlap. Counselling can help children through each of these stages (Balk, 1993, Coles, 1990, Stevens, 1998). Adults should continue to realize that the death of a parent or loved one is very painful to a child.

Betty Davies, investigator for British Columbia Research Institute for Child and Family Health, and Brenda Eng, founding director of Canuck Place Children's Hospice in Vancouver, wrote about special bereavement issues in dealing with grieving children (Davies and

Eng, 1998). They present a mnemonic to help children cope with grief within the phrase "Remember the CHILD." Recalling each letter in the word CHILD is helpful when counselling a child who is grieving.

- C is for CONSIDER. Davies and Eng call upon health care providers to treat each child as unique and not as any child or a little adult. Each child has his or her own unique concerns and a special relationship to the person who died.
- H is for HONESTY. Children can sense when adults are avoiding issues. Health providers ought to keep any discussion about death simple, use the word "death, and not avoid difficult topics.
- I is for INVOLVE. The child needs to know what is happening to the dying person and why the person is dying. A child who wants to say good-bye to the dying person and attend the funeral should be allowed to do so. Of course, a child should never be forced to do anything against his or her own will.

    L.L. de Veber, international pioneer in palliative pediatric care, emeritus professor in Pediatrics at the University of Western Ontario, and president of the de Veber Institute for Bioethics and Social Research in Toronto, concurs. He believes that "children should even be encouraged to go [to funerals], as they will regret not going for the rest of their lives and may be angry with their parents." De Veber believes that those caring for a child after a death should involve the child because he has observed that the children of dying adults are frequently neglected by hospitals and cancer clinics (De Veber, 2001, personal communication).
- L is for LISTEN. Adults must listen to the concerns of children; they should never cut them off, even if the topic is difficult for everyone involved to discuss. Adults should also help children to identify some of their own feelings, including anger and sadness, and to express those feelings in creative outlets such as art, drawing, and stories. Those caring for children need to listen carefully for any suicidal thoughts and inappropriate guilt that children might express. They should provide reassurance, explaining that the child's actions or thoughts cannot and did not cause the death.
- D is for DO IT OVER AND OVER AGAIN. One discussion of the event is not enough (Davies and Eng, 1998). Children will not engage in grief work without permission and role models. When adults talk to children honestly, and as often as necessary, about death and their honest emotions, children learn to deal with their own grief.

A member of the health-care team can teach the mnemonic "Remember the CHILD" to the parents and caregivers of a child who is mourning, to help the child deal with grief.

HOW A CHILD DEALS WITH HIS OR HER OWN DEATH

Parents learn a lot from their children about coping with life.
Muriel Spark, *The Comforters*, 1957

Everyone is saddened by the death of a child. Friends, acquaintances, and family mourn the loss of a child, while regretting deeply that the life of the child, who had so much potential, has been cut short. While the child is still alive, however, adults need to be aware of what that child feels when facing death.

The authors found very little written about how children cope with or feel about a life-threatening illness. There is much more research on how parents cope and on helping parents cope. There is even more research on how children cope with the death of a parent or a sibling than there is on how they cope with their own imminent deaths.

Should children be told they are dying? Many doctors think they are sparing the child suffering by withholding such information from them, but this is usually not true. By withholding information, physicians often contribute to a child's confusion and can actually increase physical and emotional suffering during an illness.

Myra Bluebond-Langer conducted a survey of 40 children with leukemia between the ages of 18 months and 14 years. She discovered that, regardless of well-meaning adults, children become aware of their illness and impending death on their own. In her book *The Private World of Dying Children* (1978), Bluebond-Langer identified a five-stage model of discovery.

Stage 1: Children learn they have serious illnesses. Children realize they are ill when the behavior of parents and other adults changes after their diagnosis is made. Erma Bombeck confirms Bluebond-Langer's point when she describes this stage in her book *I Want to Grow Hair, I Want to Grow Up, I Want to Go to Boise.* She writes that although the children she interviewed did not know what illness they had, they felt their family members had lined up to join what she called "The Guilt Olympics." All the adults blamed themselves for the children's diseases. These children also noticed family members whispering about their illness, without actually naming the illness. The children took their cues from their parents and other adults; they noticed changes in how adults behaved and reacted towards them. On their own, they discerned that something was wrong.

Children are very intuitive. They can often figure out that they are very ill. They notice a parent's tears or worried looks or hear their whispers. They talk to other children or adolescents. They may even read their own medical chart if it is available to them. What they believe is happening may be worse than reality. What can physicians do to help? First, they can explain the illness. They may want to use a doll, pictures, an educational video, a movie, or a book. A doctor can ask a child what he thinks was said by the physician to make sure the child understands correctly. The doctor can then clarify any misconceptions. To find out what the child knows, a doctor can ask what she thinks is happening and then invite her to ask questions and allay her fears. Sometimes a doctor can help just by listening, letting a child cry, or simply holding a hand.

JS was in the hospital twice as a child; she had a workup for epilepsy and a tonsillectomy. Her experiences taught her some good and bad ways to tell a child he or she is ill and needs treatment. The tonsillectomy was emotionally painless. The doctor, prior to surgery, explained the surgery and what was about to happen. He assured JS that she could live without her tonsils and allowed her to visit the hospital, see the surgery room, and talk to other children who had had their tonsils taken out. Consequently, even though she was only six, she wasn't afraid. She even looked forward to the ice cream promised after surgery. She knew her throat would be sore but she didn't care.

For the epilepsy workup, JS, then eight years old, was put in a hospital room with adults. No one told her what was happening or what to expect. She was terrified, especially at night after her parents went home. She also decided during the workup that she wanted to become a doctor – and a doctor who would never treat patients the way the cold and uncommunicative neurologist had treated her. She wanted to be a doctor who would listen to patients, especially children, and help them handle their fears.

Stage 2: Children learn about medication and their side effects.
This stage begins during the first treatment of the disease. Children learn about and experience the side effects of treatment, but also feel better physically because of the medications. They view themselves as "seriously ill, but likely to get better."

Emma Bombeck wrote that the worst side effect for children is what she calls the "chemo cut." She explains: "to many children of cancer, the loss of hair though chemo treatment is the final blow of indignity, the last layer of veneer that is stripped away, leaving them naked and vulnerable to society. They have lost their place in a world where peer pressure lets you in – or keeps you out" (Bombeck, 1989: 42). Children deal with the hair loss by wearing scarves, hats, wigs, and by developing funny answers. When someone asked what happened to his hair, one boy answered, "I just joined the Marines." Another would answer, "the wind just blew it out" (Bombeck, 1989: 44).

How can physicians help children at this stage? They can tell children what to expect. They can be honest with them. Children need to know that chemotherapy may cause their hair to fall out or make them nauseous. A television film about children with cancer shows a boy of seven getting a bone marrow biopsy done. He is screaming to his doctor, "I will never trust you again. This hurts." The procedure would probably still have hurt even if his doctor had told him it would be painful, but the boy would not have felt betrayed.

Another film, *My Friend Has Leukemia*, was made at Michigan State University by Robert Wilks to show elementary students what their friends with leukemia went through at the hospital when being treated for the disease. One procedure shown is bone marrow biopsy. The leukemia patients who appeared in the movie, according to Wilks, were only able to see and understand what had been done to them during the bone marrow biopsy when they saw the film; they were amazed by what they saw. If an educational video of a procedure exists, doctors could show children the film before beginning a procedure in order to lessen their fears somewhat.

Stage 3: Children concentrate on the purpose of treatment and procedures. This stage begins after the first relapse. The children begin to view themselves as "always ill, but likely to get better."

They view the treatment as a major event in their lives but continue in their normal routine whenever possible. John Gunther's book *Death Be Not Proud* provides an example of this, because he includes the diary his son kept while receiving treatment for brain cancer. In the diary his son wrote that he was studying physics and literature. He was also learning about his treatment, including what it cost. Bombeck quotes "Susan," who had liver cancer and many large scars on her abdomen. When her kindergarten friends asked her about them, she replied, "Oh, I was wounded in the war, and what a war it was."

What can doctors do at this stage? They can begin by knowing that children often ask tough questions. Because children tend to be more honest and straightforward than adults and are not yet aware of all the social taboos, they ask about what is on their minds. They may, for example, ask about another child who died and why he died. A doctor will find such a question very hard to answer if the child and the patient who died have the same illness. The child may also ask about life after death, what if feels like to die, and what happens after death. In order to be well prepared, doctors may want to think ahead of time about what they want to say.

While they may not be able to answer all the questions children ask, they can listen carefully and give each child as much attention as they would an adult. Whatever they say, they must be honest, especially as children immediately pick up on dishonesty and phoniness. Physicians can certainly address any young patient's concerns about chronic illness and about the aspects of being sick that worry them. A child may ask, for example, "When can I go back to school? Will I be able to ride my bike after the operation? Will I be home in time for my birthday? Will I be bald for a long time after you cut off my hair? Will the other kids laugh at me?" Doctors can try to answer all such questions, honestly and simply.

Doctors should also expect children to express their grief about what is happening. One patient told JS that he missed going to dances. Another said that he missed being able to walk outside and visit friends. One girl told JS she was sad about not going to her prom.

Stage 4: Children put all these pieces into a framework and see their illness as a succession of relapses and remissions. At this stage children begin to view themselves as "always ill and not likely to get better." They witness the death of other children in the hospital with them and become aware that they could die as well. They begin to have an awareness of their own mortality.

At this stage doctors should watch for emotional problems and request psychology or psychiatry consults when indicated. They might also suggest the parents talk to a counsellor.

Some children, when very sick, will not talk about dying in front of their family or friends, as they fear upsetting them. Some children may want to talk about the death of another child in the hospital, especially if the two became friends and suffered together during treatment. In doing so they are expressing their grief and may also be expressing their own fears about dying in what seems like a safe way. No one should hide the truth about what happened to the friend from the child, as that could be frightening and confusing. If appropriate, the physician might suggest to the parents of the child that he be permitted to attend the funeral of his hospital friend. A physician should remain aware that at this stage he or she may be the only person to whom child patients can or will voice their fears. If the physician finds he cannot listen, he should find someone whom the child trusts and likes and can talk to.

Stage 5: Children see death as part of the cycle. Children are aware when they are close to death. When children witness the death of another child whose illness is at the same stage as theirs, they realize they will probably die as well. From that point on, they view themselves as "dying." Their strongest desire is to keep those who love them constantly with them. Doctors should encourage the parent and children to discuss this.

In *Death Be Not Proud*, the author's 17-year old son, Johnny, writes: "Yesterday I discussed fears of death with Mother. For years I have had a lack of confidence in myself, fears about ultimate reality. Accept death with detachment. Take more pleasures in life for its own sake" (Gunther, 1949: 149).

Bluebond-Langer stated that children's strongest desire was to keep those they loved around them. John Gunther describes his son the day before he died. "But steadily he kept returning to me, as if he wanted to be particularly intimate and affectionate. All his sweetness, his remarkable goodness and pure, ineffable niceness, seemed to be bursting out of him all day" (Gunther, 1949: 107).

A child's doctor should ask, as he did in the first stages, if the child knows what is happening to her and invite questions. If possible, and with the involvement of the parents, doctors should let children decide where they want to die, if they want their favourite toy, a security blanket, or a special book, and, most important, whom they want with them. Their mother, father, a special friend or nurse? Children should be given all the time they need to say goodbye to their mother, father, and siblings. (Being able to say goodbye to their sibling(s) will help the children who are left behind deal with their grief as well.) If the people involved are not close by, the child may want to write letters to them.

Physicians can help children by keeping them free of pain. Children can point to a sad face drawing in a visual pain scale if they are in pain. If they are not in pain, they may point to a smiling face. Physicians can help, too, by listening to family members and encouraging them to get counselling if needed.

Children may benefit from having a say in deciding when they have had enough treatment. If children are old enough to understand, they can be allowed to help decide when they want no more treatment or if they want experimental treatment. Teenagers, especially, will want to be involved in treatment decisions.

Whatever age children are and whatever their illness, they need to know their parents are on their side. JS did not blame her parents for the horrible ordeal she suffered when she underwent the epilepsy workup described above. Her mother had allowed her to decide whether she would go to the hospital. JS went to the hospital only when she was emotionally ready, after waiting about a month. If she had been forced to be in the hospital against her will, she might have lost trust in her parents and blamed them for subjecting her to what happened in the hospital. Because of her mother's wisdom, she knew her parents were on her side.

According to Bluebond-Langer, the issue in the case of children is not *to tell or not to tell*, but *when to tell*, *what to tell*, and *how to do the telling*. She found that the doctor could usually take his cues from the children themselves on all these steps.

Terminally ill children, if strong enough, according to L.L. De Veber, "often wish to visit their school for social reasons and this requires team work between the school and the treatment centre.

Sensitive teachers at the school can help siblings in other classes." After the death of the child, "classmates should be encouraged to attend the funeral or hold a memorial service for their dead classmate" if they wish (DeVeber, 2001, personal communication).

Helping children cope with a life-threatening illness and death or with the death of someone close is an emotional challenge. Medical professionals find themselves dealing with emotional parents, as well as with children facing death. These professionals need to remember that when children are dying, they often become aware of their illness and impending death on their own and then pass through stages that are specific to children. Medical staff should also remember that children mourn and understand death differently, depending on their developmental age. Much more research needs to be done on the subject of children and death, so that medical professionals can better help children face their own death or the death of those they love.

QUESTIONS FOR HEALTH CARE PROFESSIONALS

A girl of eight, who is terrified of hospitals and medical procedures, suddenly has seizures. You are afraid she may have a brain tumor. How would you handle the situation?

SAMPLE ANSWER: I would explain about the tests that were involved and would say if they were going to be painful or not. I would let her parents stay with her. I would not force anything against her will.

YOUR ANSWER:

The same young girl is found to have a brain mass. The MRI suggests a medulloblastoma, a malignant tumor, so she needs a brain biopsy. Would you tell her parents first? Would you tell the child? What would you do if the parents refused further treatment on religious grounds? If the girl were 15, would you handle the situation in another way?

SAMPLE ANSWER: I would tell the parents first. I would explain the illness to the child. If the parents refused treatment, I would talk with them with their minister present. If necessary, I would consult with the hospital's Ethics Committee. If the child were 15, I would not handle the situation differently.

YOUR ANSWER:

A five-year-old child has been in the hospital for surgical treatment of pulmonic valve stenosis. He wants to go to his kindergarten class party and is very upset that he is still in the hospital. Medically, however, he is not stable. What would you do?

SAMPLE ANSWER: I would listen and let him cry. I would acknowledge his loss and acknowledge how disappointed he feels. If possible, I would contact his kindergarten teacher and ask if he or she could come to the hospital with a few of the students and have a smaller version of their party with him.

YOUR ANSWER:

John, who is 15 and has been drinking since he was 10, is at an alcohol treatment centre. He became close friends with his roommate Mark while both were at the centre. After Mark left the treatment centre, he relapsed and was killed in an auto accident while driving drunk. Should you tell John his friend is dead? Will it affect his recovery for the worse? Should you allow him to go to the funeral?

SAMPLE ANSWER: I would tell John about his friend's death or have one of the counsellors do so. John will need to get help in order to grieve and understand what happened in a way that helps his recovery. I would allow him to go to the funeral with supervision.

YOUR ANSWER:

Bobby, six, has Burkitt's lymphoma. He has already had intensive chemotherapy, after which he went into a short remission. He then had a bone marrow transplant, which his body now appears to be rejecting. He asks you if he is dying and what it will be like. His parents do not want him to know he is dying. He is obviously afraid. What do you say to him?

SAMPLE ANSWER: I would tell him that we all die sometime, but that today we have medicines that make dying painless. I would encourage the parents to talk to a chaplain or counsellor about how to communicate to their child regarding his illness.

YOUR ANSWER:

9

The Spiritual Needs of Children
Who Are Dying

You look at the sky, and you wonder what's up there, except what we see, the sun, and the moon, and the stars. Anything else? Who knows? Not me! Most of the time, I'm just going from minute to minute ... It's when something unexpected happens that I stop myself and ask what's going on: What's it all about?

Eric, 12. Robert Coles, *The Spiritual Life of Children*

L.L. (Barrie) de Veber suggested that a chapter of this book be devoted to the spiritual needs of children who are dying. He believes, as do the authors, that the physician and health care team must look after children as a whole, because sick children are more than just their physical illness (de Veber, L.L., 2001, personal communication). In this chapter we consider spirituality and how it differs from religion. We will also discuss the spiritual needs of children and how children develop spirituality over their life span. Finally, we will address how health care professionals can help children meet their spiritual needs.

What is spirituality? *The International Work Group on Death, Dying and Bereavement* of which de Veber was a member, defines it as follows: "Spirituality is concerned with the transcendental, inspirational, existential way to live one's life as well as, in a fundamental and profound sense, with the person as a human being" (Corr et al., 1993: 33).

Registered nurse Martha Farrar Highfield, while associate chief for the Nursing Service for Education at the Veterans Administration Medical Center in Los Angeles, gave the following definition of spirituality in her article "Spiritual Health of Oncology Patients:"

The spiritual dimension of persons can be uniquely defined as the human capacity to transcend self, which is phenomenologically reflected in three basic spiritual needs: (a) the need for self acceptance, a trusting relationship with self based on a sense of meaning and purpose in life; (b) the need for relationships with others and/or a supreme other (e.g. God), characterized by non-conditional love, trust, and forgiveness; and (c) the need for hope, which is the need to imagine and participate in the enhancement of a positive future. (Highfield, 1992: 2)

Each person has a life force or essence. Others sense a person's being when someone is alive; in death they see a body but do not feel a presence. Each child's values, personality, and approach to life are part of that child's spiritual being. When a child is dying, caregivers can protect, mend, and nourish the child's spiritual needs, while they care for the child.

SPIRITUALITY IS NOT THE SAME AS RELIGION

A child (indeed anyone) can be spiritual but not be religious. Spirituality is the inner dimension that gives meaning to a person's life. Many individuals depend on an organized religion to realize their spiritual selves.

Robert Coles interviewed hundreds of children so that he could understand their spiritual life. In his book *The Spiritual Life of Children* (1990) he explained the difference between religion and spirituality when he wrote:

One of our sons [made] this considered assertion: "There's religion and there's the spirit." Whence that idea? Our ten-year-old answered, "St. Paul talked about the 'letter and the spirit,' the difference, and the teacher said you can go to church all the time and obey every [church] law, and you're not really right in what you do, you're not spiritual." We asked him how we could know if we were being spiritual, not just religious, and he promptly said, "It's up to God to decide, not us." (Coles, 1990: xvii)

Religion is a vehicle that can give formal structure and direction to a child's life. Joshua, who had had his bar mitzvah three weeks before Coles interviewed him for his book, explains how his Jewish religion provides him with a structure by which to live his life:

Once you know your religion, you know how to live the way you should live, and you'll be a good person. You'll live according to the rules; and then

others will respect you and look up to you. That's important – if others respect
you. Benethon [his teacher] says if your neighbours "hold you up as wise and
good," then you're the biggest success in the world. (Coles, 1990: 266)

Because spirituality is intangible, it is hard to describe. In contrast,
because organized religions are vehicles with rules and regulations that
help one become more spiritual, they can be described. R. Twycross
(1988), a British expert on pain control and palliative care, explains
how he views the difference between spirituality and religion:

The spiritual component of a personality is the dimension or function that
integrates all other aspects of personhood. This relates to a concern with
the ultimate issues in life principles and is often seen as a search for meaning in a person's life (Why me? Why him?). Not to be confused with religion or religious, which is the practical expression of spirituality through
a framework of beliefs often actively pursued in rituals and other religious
practises. Everyone has a spiritual component, but not everyone is religious
(Twycross, 1988: 296)

THE CHILD'S DEVELOPMENTAL STAGES
OF THE CONCEPT OF DEATH

In his chapter "The Psychological Adaptation of the Dying Child,"
in the *Oxford Textbook of Palliative Medicine* (1998), Michael Stevens draws upon the work of developmental psychologist Jean Piaget
to develop a model of death awareness, with recommendations to
caregivers of dying children and adolescents.

During the first developmental stage, which lasts from birth until
the age of two, the child's intelligence consists only of sensory and
motor actions. The child has no conscious thought, a limited com-
mand of language, no concept of reality, and no concept of death.
The caregiver should provide maximum physical relief and comfort
to a child of this age who has an illness.

During the second developmental stage, which lasts from early
childhood through middle childhood until adolescence, the child's
understanding develops. From two years until seven years of age,
the child's thinking is egocentric and magical. The child perceives
death as reversible, as a temporary restriction, departure, or sleep.

The child, then, may expect the dead person, including himself, to return, as if from a trip. A young child who is very sick may worry about being buried alive, being too cold or hot, suffocating, or not having enough to eat. The child needs assurance that none of this will happen.

Stevens recommends minimizing the child's separation from his parents when ill. He also encourages evaluating children to see if they are feeling guilt, rejection, anger, or resentment of self or others. If children feel that their bad thoughts or actions are to blame for their illness, the adult caregiver or spiritual advisor may need to correct this perception.

In middle childhood, which lasts from 7 years of age until 11 or 12 (labeled preadolescence), the child's orientation is no longer centered on the ego. The child's thinking is limited to the actual features, though they may be absent, of a situation rather than to abstract relationships and hypotheses. The child understands the principles of conservation and reversibility but is not capable of abstract reasoning. The child at this age sees death as irreversible but capricious.

Stevens recommends that the caregiver or spiritual counsellor of a terminally ill child evaluate possible fears of abandonment, destruction, and body mutilation. He encourages the caregiver to be truthful and open, to provide details about treatments, and to foster the child's sense of control and mastery. He also advises the caregiver to make sure the child does not view the treatment as a punishment. He suggests that adults make it possible for the sick child to see his or her friends.

During the third developmental stage, which begins at 12 and continues throughout adulthood (although some adults never achieve this level of thinking), children integrate cognitive structures and functions and achieve full intellectual capacities, including the ability to deal effectively with a world of abstract ideas and hypothetical thinking. Reality is now objective.

Adolescents perceive death as irreversible, universal, and personal but distant. They view death as natural and physiological and may now have theological explanations for death. The caregiver and spiritual advisor can help by reinforcing a comfortable body image and positive self-esteem, allowing the adolescent to vent anger, providing privacy, and supporting reasonable measures for independence.

Stevens encourages the caregiver and spiritual advisor to be clear, honest, and direct. Adolescents should have access to their peers and may benefit from mutual support groups.

SPIRITUAL ISSUES OF CHILDREN

In a paper entitled "The Influence of Spirituality on Dying Children's Perceptions of Death" in *The Innocence of Childhood: Helping Children and Adolescents Cope with Life Threatening Illness and Dying* (1995), de Veber suggests the following spiritual concerns of dying children, using case vignettes that focus on the child's

- Asking "why me"?
- Hoping for a potentially spiritual experience, such as a special trip or event.
- Needing to believe in an after-life, where the child can meet others in heaven or another spiritual place.
- Wanting to know that family members, loved ones, and pets will be all right after the child has died.
- Expecting to learn more about Jesus, God, the Buddha, or the religious deity of their belief system.
- Wondering what it is like to die.
- Worrying that they have done something bad that has caused their death.

How can caregivers and spiritual advisors help children with these issues? De Veber agrees with B.J. Prescott-Erickson (1987) that the spiritual advisor should arrange a visit with the child alone and in a place where the child will be comfortable. Throughout the encounter, the advisor should be honest and direct. The advisor should explain who he is and that he is visiting to discuss spiritual concerns and needs. The advisor should guide the conversation, based on the child's responses and questions, since the child needs to set the agenda. She might ask the child how he would describe God and whether he believes that God acts in a meaningful way. If the advisor wants to pray with a terminally ill child, she should ask first if the child wants to pray and respect the child's wishes if she does not want to do so. If the child is willing to pray, the advisor should ask her what she wants to pray about. Regular follow-up visits are important (de Veber, 1995).

In the *Oxford Textbook of Palliative Medicine* (1998), in the chapter "Creative Arts and Literature," David Frampton discusses the role of a palliative-care arts program. A program can allow the child to occupy time creatively and to leave something behind. It can also improve feelings of personal worth and purpose and provide a non-threatening way to explore fears and worries. A staff member can ask the child to explain his or her creation in order to obtain insight into the child's spiritual and psychological well-being.

Music therapy, according to Stevens (1998), is also a useful tool. A variety of techniques are available, including song writing and selection, lyric substitution, improvisation, and guided imagery. All of these techniques can be used to encourage the child to release his or her fears and express religious feelings.

If a child has questions about death, reading can open up discussion. Stevens recommends the following books:

Alcott, L.M. *Little Women* (there are many editions)
Berstein, J.E. and S.V. Gullo. 1977. *When People Die*. New York: Dutton
Bleeker, Z. 1970. *Life and Death*. New York: Morrow
Fassler, J. 1971. *My Grandpa Died Today*. New York: Human Sciences Press
Grollman, E.A. 1976. *Talking About Death – A Dialogue Between Parent and Child*. Boston: Beacon Press
White, E.B. 1952. *Charlotte's Web*. (many editions)
Bleeker, Z. 1970. *Life and Death*. New York: Morrow.

Often a dying child can find comfort in the religious traditions and the rites of their faith. Robert Coles describes how Leah, who was about 11 years old at her death, found comfort in her religion.

I remember my last visit to Leah. She was not far from death. Her body had withered; she was jaundiced, dehydrated, sweaty, and feverish. At her bedside was her father's Bible ... I saw in Leah a child intensely attached to a family's religious and spiritual life, its prayers and food and ceremonies, its spoken acknowledgement of the Lord, its remembrance of His words, of what He and His people had experienced together in the past and were still in that hospital room, in our time, undergoing together. "I'd like to go to that 'high rock,'" Leah told her dad just before she slipped into a final coma – and from then until her death, her heartbroken but proud and strong father could be heard by nurses and doctors and ward helpers and visitors and family members saying in Hebrew the 61st Psalm: "Hear my cry, O God; attend unto my prayer. From the end of the earth will I cry unto thee, when my heart is overwhelmed: lead me to the rock that is higher than I." The rock for Leah, for their family, was a Judaism that would not break or yield, even at the death of a young girl (Coles, 1990: 276).

All children have a spiritual dimension when they near death or cope with a life-threatening illness. They ask many questions such as "Why me? Why am I here? What will happen to my loved ones and me when I die? Do I matter?" While the spiritual needs of dying children are those of all children regardless of health, they also include spiritual needs that arise because they are reacting to illness or facing death. Health care providers and spiritual advisors who understand the child's symbolic language and take into account developmental levels and experiences can help children address their spiritual needs at this painful time. Many tools exist, including music therapy, art therapy, religious rituals, and the assistance of spiritual leaders. Above all, all the involved adults must be there for children and listen to them.

10

Physicians as Patients

Now this young guy, thirty years my junior, had the temerity to raise the possibility of cancer. What right did he have to do that? I'm the doctor. I tell people they have cancer, but no one says that to me. Doctors are immune; they don't get sick.

Edward E. Rosenbaum, *The Doctor*, 1991

Joan Lawrence, a psychiatrist in Queensland, Australia, and past president of the Royal Australian and New Zealand College of Psychiatrists, observes that physicians and their patients share a belief that doctors are superhuman, invulnerable to the ills of mankind, and thus immortal. Patients would like to believe that their doctors are never ill. Both doctors and patients alike are upset when a physician is sick. Lawrence cites the example of a colleague who, six months after his forty-ninth birthday, had a crushing pain in the centre of his chest. He ignored the pain for three days, even though his father had died suddenly of a myocardial infarction at the age of 50. He only decided to seek help after he experienced severe pain while walking up a flight of stairs. His patients were very upset; one even stated that he had no right to be ill.

Lawrence believes that significant problems arise when the doctors change their role, becoming patients instead of doctors. Patient-doctors are not always dealt with appropriately. The treating doctor may talk to the patient-doctor as if seeking a second opinion from a colleague, thereby encouraging the patient-doctor to deny that he is a patient. In this situation the treating doctor may accept the patient-doctor's diagnosis and so may not perform a thorough physical or take a good history. The treating doctor is then likely to miss the true diagnosis. The treating doctor may also want to deny the seriousness of the patient-doctor's illness because of his own denial and avoidance defenses. After all, if this doctor can become ill, so can he. In some situations the treating physician may not explain the illness or treatments completely, because she has an unrealistic expectation about the patient-doctor's clinical knowledge of the illness (Lawrence, 1989). All of the above can lead to inferior or incomplete care of the patient-doctor.

As patients, physicians have some special needs, simply because of the nature of the profession. They certainly need privacy. Although this should go without saying, it is often ignored. The authors have seen the boundary crossed on more than one occasion. Most of these boundary violations occur when physicians are patients in the hospitals in which they work. Physicians and staff who are not assigned to the patient's case may check charts and case files, convincing themselves that doing so is acceptable because the doctor is a staff member.

Of course, doing this is completely unacceptable. A physician or nurse/patient deserves the same privacy as any other patient. Because a member of a hospital staff knows a patient-doctor personally does not entitle him to look at the patient's personal medical history. Only those assigned to the case have the right to read the files.

Another problem arises when members of the medical team, especially the physician, do not provide the same personal and compassionate touch to a patient-doctor that they would to other patients. They may think that, because of her medical knowledge, the patient-doctor does not need such consideration. However, simply because physicians know the technical ins and outs of their medical problem does not make them immune to the concerns and fears of other patients. They need the same kindness and attention as any other patient.

JS has had several physician friends who had AIDS and were frightened that they would die from the illness in the same way their own patients had died. They needed reassurance. JS understood this, in part because she had once developed a severe pneumonia, which could not be identified. She was quite fearful when told she needed a bronchoscopy, because a patient had a respiratory arrest during the first bronchoscopy she witnessed as a medical student. She was relieved that the physician allowed her to express her fear. She was then sedated and nothing went wrong during the procedure.

Probably all doctors have been frightened by medical procedures, such as spinal taps and bone marrow aspirations. Sometimes physicians and nurses fear such procedures because they know just what can go wrong and are well aware of the pain and discomfort involved. Because they may know too much for their own good, they need members of their medical team to recognize that their expertise and knowledge may make them especially fearful. Patient-doctors may know, for example, that pancreatic cancer has a poor prognosis. If they think this is what they have, they may not want to find out. Physicians caring for physicians need to be aware that their patients may possess more knowledge than they are able to handle emotionally.

Physicians who are patients also need a full disclosure of their illness and the available treatment. While doctor-patients may be experts in their own medical specialty, they may not be highly versed in the area in which they're seeking help and treatment. When treating other physicians, doctors may tend to assume that they do not need to explain anything because the patient-doctors already know what is going on. Physicians need to provide doctor-patients with the full and complete information every patient needs.

One of the physicians with AIDS, mentioned above, became very ill after treating many HIV patients. He told JS he was glad to hand over his care to another physician because he was tired of keeping up with all the new information. He also wanted the comfort of another person caring for him. At the same time, he wanted his physician to explain all the treatment options to him.

Physicians are not immune to serious illness and death. If they become patients, they deserve the same privacy that all patients do. Their physicians should be as kind to them as they are to their other patients. These physicians must also be thorough when giving their doctor-patients physicals and taking their histories to avoid a mistaken diagnosis. Physicians must provide complete information about the nature of the illness and treatment options, realizing that a patient-doctor may not know much about his or her illness.

QUESTIONS FOR HEALTH CARE PROFESSIONALS

As a physician, how would you want to be treated if you checked into a hospital for needed treatment?

SAMPLE ANSWER: I would be concerned that I wouldn't receive the best of care since my colleagues would be too embarrassed to provide me with complete information or would assume that I already knew certain things about my condition. Because of this, I would go to a hospital where no one knew me.

YOUR ANSWER:

PART THREE

Coping

11

Coping with the Death of a Patient

Neither the sun nor death can be looked at steadily.
                    Francois de la Rochefoucauld (1613-1680), *Maxims*

We see the world piece by piece, as the sun, the moon,
the animal, the tree; but not the whole, of which these are the
shining parts.
                    Ralph Waldo Emerson (1803–1882), *The Over-Soul*

The word compassion, which means "to suffer with," comes from two Latin roots, *com* and *passion*. When physicians feel compassion, they often bear a very heavy personal cost. When physicians open their eyes to death and grief, they may become aware, like the patient and family, of their own mortality. They may also realize their limitations as healers and remember their past or threatened losses.

Many doctors deal with death by not becoming involved with their patients. In doing so, they deny themselves a richer perspective on life. As Richard Edlich and Elisabeth Kübler-Ross explained in an article titled *"On Death and Dying in the Emergency Department:"*

When we view the shadow of death, we face our own mortality and appreciate that life is finite. The dying person develops deeper meanings and priorities for his life, because he can no longer postpone opportunities. Consequently, he must make the most of every minute. Health professionals who care for the dying patient have the unrivaled opportunity to examine what makes life meaningful. As we share our insights on dying, we fortuitously discover the joys of unconditional love in a glorious journey through life. For many physicians, problems of living become so complicated and overwhelming that this contemplation of our death may serve as an emotional rebirth, revitalizing ambitions and passions, and bringing to our lives new dimensions and meanings. (Edlich and Kübler-Ross, 1992: 228–9)

In a study of 49 hospice medical directors, 16 per cent of the physicians reported suicidal thoughts that lasted more than two weeks, while 8 per cent admitted to suicidal thoughts that lasted less than two weeks (Vachon, 1995). Feelings of grief among health practitioners can appear in the following or other forms:

• Anticipatory grief, which occurs while the patient is still living but the physician begins to withdraw emotionally
• Denial of grief and inability to show grief, which manifests itself when physicians refuse to react to the death of patients
• Masked grief, in which the physician becomes physically ill or engages in risky behavior as a substitute for grief.
  (Vachon, 1995).

The fears of physicians are related to their attitudes about informing dying patients of their condition. Physicians who believe that patients "should never be made aware that they are dying" tend to feel greater fear about their own death and hold more rigid attitudes about treating terminal patients (Barroso et al., 1992). In reality, they sometimes hear about death within their own ranks.

Recently, a young surgeon whom the authors knew and his daughter died in a car wreck. This surgeon was handsome, energetic, and humorous, the last person anyone expected to die. On learning of his death, both authors thought, "This really makes you stop and think how unpredictable and fragile life is." The death of another physician hits very close to home.

The authors asked physicians and registered nurses how the death of patients affect them, how they cope, and how they take care of their own needs at these times. Nurse practitioner Tina Martin responded:

It depends on the patient, of course. When the patient has died in a manner in which they felt comfortable and accepted, it's easier, but it is still sad. When the system does not allow this, I get angry. If the relationship to the patient was close, I feel the loss of knowing that person. I feel every person I meet affects my life in some way. I say goodbye in my own way. Sometimes it has been at the bedside. Other times it has been at a ceremony. I always acknowledge saying goodbye and letting go with some sort of ritual. Sometimes I journal briefly in my mind or on paper. With a colleague, I review the care given the patient. I see if there's something I could have done differently and learn from it. I thank the person for being a part of my life. Then I let it go. I do not blame myself or the patient for dying. I know I have no control over things. I make sure I use a large part of my life to enjoy living, doing things I enjoy.

Fran Blais, an infectious disease physician, answered:

It depends on how long I have followed the patient and the relationship that develops. It is also age-dependent. The younger and the more close the relationship, the more unexpected, the more personal it is to me. It always creates a sense of helplessness. I've been able to handle my own needs upon the death of a patient through conversations with my colleagues and spouse. I vent. I get it out. In addition, I have developed my own routines to deal with stress – hobbies, exercise, and reading.

A family physician who is living with AIDS tried to learn from the death of a patient: "I feel the individual loss. I always seem to review the process and look for places where I could have intervened further or not at all."

Brady Allen, a respected AIDS physician in Dallas, Texas, has found that ignoring the death of a patient causes even greater stress than facing emotions:

It depends on my own emotional investment with each particular patient. Some patients' deaths don't have much effect at all while others provoke sadness, loss, and grieving. I try to think over and talk about each death and what it means to me. I have found that if I ignore a death, my stress level and anger level rise significantly. Sometimes I go to funerals, but that's infrequent. In psychotherapy, both group and individual, I acknowledge each death and talk about it with others. I usually send a sympathy card to the family and significant other. As best I can, I try to stay physically and emotionally fit.

The authors noticed that most of the medical professionals who responded to their questions felt a degree of grief that was directly related to how close they felt to a particular patient and family. This was especially true in emergency situations, when the traumatic nature of the situation causes those involved to bond quickly.

The authors also noted a wide variety of responses. An angry addictionologist said he believes that death is so much stronger than doctors are and feels at times that "medicine is such a sham." Nurse practitioner Martin, on the other hand, appears to accept death and her lack of control over it.

The responses also indicated a wide range of coping skills. Some doctor and nurse respondents admitted they talked to no one and did little to care for themselves. Others, however, realized the emotional impact of death and took good care of themselves; hobbies, rituals, therapy groups, and exercise helped them reenergize and restore themselves.

QUESTIONS FOR HEALTH CARE PROFESSIONALS

After answering the questions below, the authors encourage medical professionals to read their responses again at a later time. Those who fail to care for themselves might jot down a few suggestions about how they might begin to do so. These suggestions will be useful later in the book, when the authors ask medical professionals to design a specific plan of self-care that will meet their needs.

How are you affected by the death of a patient?

SAMPLE ANSWER: Sometimes I feel guilty because I wonder if I could have done more. I always feel sad for the patient and the family. If the patient was someone I especially enjoyed seeing, I will miss their presence in my office.

YOUR ANSWER:

How do you cope when your patient dies? How do you care for your own needs at these times?

SAMPLE ANSWER: I talk to a friend or colleague about my feelings. I send a condolence card to the family or attend the funeral if the patient was someone I was close to. I take some time to think about the patient.

YOUR ANSWER:

PHYSICIANS DESCRIBE HOW THEY TALK TO PATIENTS

The authors learned much from the way physicians talk to other medical professionals, patients, and their families about dealing with the subjects of death and dying. The doctors who responded suggested that physicians need to express their feelings and emotions. An internist wrote: "Communicate your feelings to patients – if you're afraid, say it. At the same time, have the patient explain what they are feeling as well. You need open communication, eye contact, support, and a proper amount of empathy."

Of course, doctors should first understand their feelings, before expressing them to patients or their families. If they fail to do so, they may be caught unprepared, so that they say things they do not really mean or that may cause harm. Also, if doctors understand their feelings, they may avoid talking about subjects such as life after death, which are better left to other professionals.

An infectious disease physician practising in Fort Worth, Texas, wrote: "You should learn and analyze your own feelings regarding death. Develop a comfort with the process. Educate yourself by reading as much on the topic as you can. Offer advice, but don't carry the therapy too far. Remember, this is a time for support, gentleness, and handholding. As much as possible, focus on listening and remaining quiet. Remember, this is about the patient's and family's agenda, not yours."

A registered nurse emphasized that medical professionals need to listen and to disregard their own agendas. She said:

Respect the fact that it is not your life and death. It is the patient's. Honestly, share what you know and defer on what you do not know. Allow the patient to make as many choices as he or she wishes. Give as much control to them as possible. If requested by the patient, make use of family and friends. And call on other professionals for help if you need to. This is no time for territorializing and claims of ownership. Your job is to listen to the patient's fears and hopes and act accordingly.

Probably the most sage advice of all is to simply be there and provide comfort. One physician wrote: "My uncle died in 1995. My family and friends wanted questions answered. They were hoping for another opinion, I believe. But I also think people benefit simply from another person's presence, their willingness to talk and just be there."

A hospice worker who responded to the authors' study echoed these sentiments: "Don't be afraid to know your patients who have a terminal illness. Share your time and listen to them. In working with hospice patients, I have come in contact with many who have never had the opportunity to discuss their terminal illness with their physician. Most patients respect their physician and have a need to feel the physician is involved in their care."

Still another physician wrote: "As they are capable, allow patients to experience the process of dying. Offer yourself as comfort and keep family and friends apprised of the situation in order to avoid surprises and to ease the transition once the patient has died. Let the family know that there is no proper way to mourn and not to stifle their grief. This grief, and the pain that accompanies it, is usually equal to the love that was shared."

REVIEWING THE STAGES OF DYING: SUGGESTIONS ON HOW TO DEAL WITH DYING PATIENTS

Based on the communications of physicians and health-care professionals and their experiences over the years, the authors offer the guidelines below. Their suggestions for helping the dying patients and their families are organized according to the six stages of dying presented earlier in the book.

Stage One: Recognition

Recognition occurs when patients know their life is approaching its end. That moment may occur when a person comes face to face with terminal illness. At that point, attitudes, actions, perspectives, goals, and relationships all change. It's a brand new situation for the patient.

The situation changes for physicians as well. How does a doctor tell a patient she has a terminal illness? How does a doctor tell someone else he has less than a year to live? A doctor can:

- Determine the patient's illness and explain it in an understandable way. At this stage, patients don't care about their doctors' medical expertise. They want to know the basics. Since doctors spend so much time with their colleagues, they tend to lapse into jargon. This is not the time to do that. As bearers of a very disturbing message, doctors need to speak as simply as possible.
- Find an appropriate time and place to tell the person. This is not always easy to determine. If a doctor says she will call a patient when the test results come in, she should call and ask the patient to come to her office or meet in a neutral spot that the patient chooses. Some patients may want the news immediately, over the phone. This is not the best way to provide news, especially if the patient is alone at home as he will then have no one to offer support.

  Also, when a patient hears bad news on the phone, she does not see her doctor's expressions or body language. A doctor might fail to convey what he really feels on the phone, perhaps seeming cold, although his expression would have revealed his real concern. Doctors may lose information that a patient is providing as well. A patient may say he is fine with the news, while his body language shows he is devastated. One patient, upon learning of a recurrence of her breast cancer, became extremely anxious and in need of much reassurance. Another patient thought her doctor had said she had cancer, when that is not what the doctor said at all. It's always better for a doctor to deliver information about an illness in person.

- Allow patients to ask questions in their own way. Some patients ask many questions because of their anxiety and fear. Their doctors should allow them to do this; even if the questions seem irrational, asking them may be very important to the patient. Other patients respond to bad news with only a stunned silence. Their doctors should sit, remaining silent too. They should also encourage any family members who are present to honour the silence. After an appropriate amount of time, doctors can then ask their patients if they have any questions. After patients have asked them, the family members may ask their own.
- Let their patients know that they will remain in contact. Since doctors bring the news of a serious illness to a patient, their patients will turn to them for more information or to ask questions later. Doctors should let their patients know that they will remain available to answer any of those questions.
- Make arrangements for counselling. Doctors can let patients who are unusually anxious, depressed, or overwhelmed know that they and their family members might benefit from a few sessions with a licenced psychologist or psychiatrist who specializes in psychological factors in medical illnesses. Doctors may make professional referrals or, when appropriate, refer patients to good free or low cost services. Doctors may also suggest that patients who are already seeing a psychologist or psychiatrist continue to do so.

In an excellent article, "Ten Commandments for the Care of Terminally Ill Patients," psychiatrist James Whitten (1998) recommends that doctors:

- Be honest. They should offer only as much help as patients request, asking if patients would like to hear the information or would prefer a family member be told.
- Bring in other specialists. They can suggest medical, psychiatric, surgical, or other consultations early on.

- Not abandon their patients when they leave the hospital. Primary physicians should not sign off on a case because a patient goes to a hospice or nursing home. Instead they should continue to spend some time with the patient and family.
- Stay in regular contact with the patient. Because their visits are still valuable, doctors should not make fewer or shorter visits to dying patients. Patients and families are very aware of any changes in a doctor's routine and may perceive it as abandonment.
- Seek emotional support from peers and family. Doctors may discuss their feelings about their patients with their own spouses or families and with other physicians, nurses, and staff at the nursing station, in the physicians' lounge, or the surgical dressing room. Because doctors must observe privacy and confidentiality laws when talking about patients with those who are not directly involved, they must be careful not to provide identifying information.
- Talk with the patient's family. Doctors can ask if the family will appoint one person with whom they can communicate regularly. They can expect that family member to be angry, depressed, guilty, or fearful of the medical surrounding. When talking to the appointed family member, doctors should not use any jargon.
- Treat the patient as a valuable human being. Doctors must remember that quality of life is important even when near death. Sometimes "a cure is not the objective and our goal is to help the patient remain a human being during the process of dying."
- Try to maintain hope. Most patients hope for a cure, so when they ask how long they have left, their doctors should not make their situations sound completely hopeless.
(Whitten, 1998)

Stage Two: The Process of Dying

As an illness worsens, patients will begin to experience the physical and emotional consequences of deterioration. Once this begins, doctors may wish to:

- Monitor arrangements for medicine and pain control.
- Continue to provide treatment and to make referrals to specialists as needed. Doctors can tell patients, who are going through many emotional changes and adjustments at this point, about any new

treatments that are available or will soon be available. They ought to allow patients to change their treatment levels.

- Discuss the fears of their patients. Patients are often very frightened at this stage. Even if doctors can do nothing, they can listen to their patients express their feelings.
- Help locate the necessary community resources needed by the patient. With the help of social workers, doctors may help patients find the many and varied services available to them. A patient who is alone might need to find a companion, while another may need to consult a service that provides legal and financial advice to patients and families.
- Discuss where the patient would like to die. Some patients may choose to die at home with hospice care. Under some conditions, however, they may be unable to receive all the care they need in a hospice situation. Doctors can also discuss whether patients want to become organ donors.

Stage Three: The Moment of Death and
Stage Four: Departure of the Spirit or Life Force

When doctors sense patients do not have much longer to live, they should notify the family that death is imminent. They should also honour the wishes of patients who have requested DNR status. At this point doctors may:

- Arrange for a spiritual advisor to be present. If the patient and family have arranged for a spiritual advisor to be present, someone in the medical staff may need to contact that individual.
- Respect the patient's belief system. Doctors may also need to ask family members to respect the patient's belief system, if their own differs. If they fail to do so when necessary, the patient will suffer. If appropriate, doctors may also pray for their patients.

Stage Five: Terminal Care of the Body

The medical staff must do its best to facilitate and honour the religious customs of the patient. (For example, in some instances the burial must take place very quickly.) The doctor or a member of the medical staff will:

- Be sure that tubes and other external devices are removed from the body. Family members often want to see a loved one as remembered, so it is important to remove devices from the patient and medical equipment from the area around the patient.
- Allow the family to be alone with the patient.
- Arrange for an autopsy if the family or patient has requested it when required by law.
- Arrange for respectful transport of the body.

Stage Six: Dealing with Grief and Loss

After a patient has died, a caring doctor will:

- Talk to the family and friends of patients. Family members are coping with the unreality of what has just happened, so they need to talk about the loss and ask questions in order to make it real. Doctors are in a unique and valuable position and so can help them grasp the details of the death. Family members also need to express their feelings – their anger, guilt, sadness, anxiety, and relief. By letting them talk and acknowledging that their feelings are normal, doctors encourage them to continue the grief work later on.
- Explain what happened at death. As the authors stated above, the family usually wants to know the causes of death and to ask other questions. When explaining, doctors should remember to speak plainly and briefly and to avoid jargon.
- Be available. Doctors can let the family know how to contact them if they have further questions or are in need of help.
- Refer family members and friends to individual or family counselling or a grief support group when appropriate. It is a good idea to be aware of grief support groups in your area so that you can make a referral. Persons or families whose loss appears to result in very difficult adjustments, such as a widow or widower whose life revolved around the deceased, will frequently need grief counselling to cope successfully with the situation. You will also want to know several therapists effective with grieving individuals and families.
- Deal with their own grief. Doctors need to acknowledge their own loss when patients die whom they knew or treated for years, liked personally, or for whom they felt responsible. Doctors, who may feel angry, sad, guilty, and helpless after a patient dies, will need

their own families, friends, and trusted colleagues to help them express their feelings.

ADDITIONAL WAYS THAT DOCTORS MAY ASSIST FAMILIES

The authors offer the following suggestions to doctors who wish to help the families of patients who have died. Because these suggestions apply to matters that are more personal than those described above, doctors may choose those that suit their temperaments, levels of comfort, and relationships with particular patients. Doctors may:

- Call and express their concern to the family, if this is done out of genuine concern rather than a sense of duty, as most families can detect the difference. Doctors may want to ask how everyone is doing if they have not heard from them a week or two after the death. At this time doctors may also ask the family members who are their patients if they need to come in for a visit.
- Attend the funeral. Some doctors even offer to speak if the family is comfortable with their doing so. Doctors should ask themselves if speaking at the funeral would help or hurt them or the patient's family.
- Send a card or flowers to the family or funeral home.
- Cultivate their listening skills. In some instances, family members may seek counsel or simply want to talk, thereby helping everyone work through grief and sorrow in his or her own way.
- Follow the suggestions in "Things to say" and "Things not to say" to bereaved family members that appear in the grief section of chapter 2 (37–8).

Because death is part of the life cycle, doctors deal with it throughout their careers. Still, learning about death is not any easier for doctors than it is for patients and their families. The authors hope that understanding the stages of death will help physicians communicate more effectively and in an open, honest, and compassionate way with those who are dying or may die and with their families and friends.

Understanding the stages of death will also help physicians face their own deaths, which they must do before they can help patients face their fears. Among the most important ways that physicians in training or practicing physicians can serve others are by:

- Discussing death and dying with patients and families
- Handling feelings associated with death – both their own and those of patients and families
- Caring for dying patients.

QUESTIONS FOR HEALTH CARE PROFESSIONALS

Remembering that practice is the building block of medicine and the six stages of dying discussed previously, how would you answer the following questions:

An 87-year-old Alzheimer's patient, who has no living will and has had a stroke, suddenly develops a pulmonary embolism. Her daughter realizes that her mother is dying but cannot bring herself to write a DNR order. What would you do?

SAMPLE ANSWER: In this situation, I would probably go ahead and do a full code because the daughter did not approve a DNR order. However, I would explain to the daughter the consequences of what she was doing and help her deal with her ambivalence and fear.

YOUR ANSWER:

A young girl dies suddenly on the tennis court of a cardiac arrest. The cause is unclear. You tried resuscitating the girl for over an hour. How do you decide whether to stop the resuscitation? Do you decide on your own to go on trying or do you involve the family in this decision?

SAMPLE ANSWER: In this situation I would explain to the family what was happening and probably go along with the family's wishes because if they felt that resuscitation had not been done long enough, they would probably feel a great deal of shame and guilt.

YOUR ANSWER:

Your patient, who was addicted to drugs or alcohol, has terminal cancer. How would you handle the patient's pain control?

SAMPLE ANSWER: Even if a person has been a drug and alcohol abuser, that person has the right to pain control and may require even more pain medicine than usual. To avoid abuse, I would probably prescribe the pain medicine for a given amount of time and refill the prescription when necessary. I would not be reluctant to treat a person with a terminal illness with pain medicine.

YOUR ANSWER:

A young woman, who presents with breast cancer that has spread to her lymph nodes, has seen a surgeon who told her that her illness was terminal. Hysterical and crying, she is in your office. How would you respond to her?

SAMPLE ANSWER: I would listen to the patient and attempt to give her hope. I would refer her to a program such as the M.D. Anderson Cancer Center, where experimental drugs are available. I'd let her know all her options. If she chose not to fight the cancer, I could accept that but would encourage her to get the maximum treatment. I would keep in contact.

YOUR ANSWER:

A 34-year-old man tests HIV positive. He has a life partner whose CD4 count is 50. What would you say to the patient?

SAMPLE ANSWER: I would tell him that HIV is now being considered a chronic disease. I would discuss treatment options. I would listen to his fears and concerns. I would start him on prophylactic medicines if indicated. I would also refer him to a social worker for counselling and plan to see him regularly.

YOUR ANSWER:

A five-year-old girl has acute leukemia. Would you tell her? What would you say to the family?

SAMPLE ANSWER: I would talk to the family first. Then I would explain the situation to the child in a language she could understand. I would arrange for treatment and see the family and child regularly, even if I were not treating the leukemia.

YOUR ANSWER:

12

Physicians' Self-Care

I am not afraid of storms, for I'm learning to sail my ship.
> Louisa May Alcott (1832–1888)

Don't compromise yourself – you're all you've got.
> Janis Joplin (1943–1970)

Hope raises its voice sometimes. It has to talk louder than fear. Sometimes you can coax it to come to you, but most of the time you have to be patient and wait. Then it will come to you.
> Erma Bombeck, *I Want to Grow Hair, I Want to Grow Up,*
> *I Want to Go to Boise: Children Surviving Cancer,* 1989

While physicians are very good at taking care of others, they often fall short when it comes to taking care of themselves. Self-care is especially important when doctors are taking care of patients who are dying or have died.

Because physicians give so much emotionally, spiritually, and physically, they also need to give back to themselves. When they become too stoic, believing they can handle everything all the time, they risk burn out and depression, become prone to substance abuse, and may shut down their emotions and feelings for the sake of others. There are times when they have to be stoic and strong: there's nothing wrong with that. If it becomes their way of life, however, not only will they suffer, so will their patients.

Physicians can do much to facilitate their self-care. Following is a brief list, which the authors will expand upon in this chapter and in chapters to follow. Physicians can:

- Nourish hope
- Maintain healthy boundaries, both professionally and personally
- Deal with the guilt and shame that may follow a patient's death or a clinical error
- Identify and seek help for clinical depression, anxiety disorders, or sleep problems
- Have regular physicals and address their medical problems with their own physicians
- Learn to express emotions and feelings in a healthy manner, individually and as part of a health care team
- Make time for relaxation and meditation each day
- Engage in regular, noncompetitive exercise
- Make time for recreational periods during the workweek and for regular vacations every few months, even if only for a few days
- Nourish their inner selves, developing their spirituality.

HOPE FOR THE HEALER

Doctors experience hope as confidence that a patient will recover. They lose that hope when they know that, despite their best efforts, some patients will not recover.

Because they care for many patients with life-threatening diseases, including advanced-stage cancer, end-stage lung disease, and drug-resistant HIV, doctors sometimes experience a sense of futility. Doctors often lose hope for their patients with terminal illnesses; at times, they may even wonder why they continue to treat them. JS remembers the deep sense of collective hopelessness that she and her colleagues felt at the 1994 International Conference on AIDS; those attending left the gathering well aware of the lack of new drugs and treatments for their patients.

So how do doctors maintain hope when dealing with a threatening or a terminal illness? Hope, to be valid, must be based on a realistic set of goals and beliefs. Otherwise, the hope is false, and that can be emotionally devastating or even fatal. Physicians can realistically hope for their patients that:

- A disease can be cured, if it is a disease like pneumonia, for which there is a cure

- A disease will go into remission, as often happens with leukemia and some other forms of cancer
- Incurable diseases, such as hypertension, HIV, and diabetes, can be controlled as chronic illnesses
- If a disease is not treatable, preventing pain and providing a better quality of life prior to death will be an important part of their care.

When no new treatments are available, or even expected, what can physicians do to remain hopeful? They can:

- Remember that patients may continue to survive with illness, for instance, long-term survivors of cancer or AIDS
- Use preventative measures such as vaccinations, healthy diets, nutrition, and prophylactic medicines to prevent infection and prolong life
- Review the medical literature, read journals, and attend conferences to see what advances have been made in treatments and medications
- Become involved in research intended to prolong the quality of life of future patients.

When a patient is not responding to treatment or further treatment appears inappropriate, doctors can revive their own hope for the patient in several specific ways. They can:

- Refer the patient to a specialty centre or to another physician for a second opinion
- Present the patient's case at Grand Rounds
- Review the medical literature for new tests or treatments
- Remember that there may be treatments available of which they are unaware
- Provide palliative care that maintains some quality of life.

In 1994, before the current drug therapies for HIV/AIDS were available, JS treated three young men for AIDS. None of these men responded to even the most aggressive, up-to-date treatments and all died with six months of each other. JS then sank into a deep state of despair. To regain some sense of hope, she read *My Life* (Ryan White, 1992) and *The Screaming Room: A Mother's Journal of Her Son's Struggle with AIDS* (Barbara Peabody, 1987). Both Ryan and

Peabody's son Peter died of AIDS-related illnesses that would have been preventable and treatable with current medications.

QUESTIONS FOR HEALTH CARE PROFESSIONALS

Which of the above suggestions would help you maintain hope for a patient in your care?

SAMPLE ANSWER: I referred my patient to the Mayo Clinic for a second surgical opinion. His current recovery from surgery for ulcerative colitis was going badly and the patient was losing hope.

YOUR ANSWER:

What else would you do?

SAMPLE ANSWER: Even though the Mayo Clinic was in another state, I kept in touch with the patient by phone as he underwent another major surgery.

YOUR ANSWER:

Have you ever felt hopeless about a patient(s)?

SAMPLE ANSWER: Yes. A patient with a low CD4 count could not tolerate any medications for HIV and was getting multiple opportunistic infections. I felt powerless to help her.

YOUR ANSWER:

What did you do to develop hope?

SAMPLE ANSWER: I referred the patient to a major research centre where clinical trials were being conducted for patients in her situation.

YOUR ANSWER:

MAINTAINING BOUNDARIES

And finally, we are powerless over other people. We can try to keep someone from dying. Ultimately, though, we have no control over other people living and dying. When we accept this, life is easier for us and for the people around us.

Perry Tilleraas, *The Color of Light*, 1988

When health care professionals maintain necessary boundaries, they can avoid unnecessary conflict and provide their patients with care that is unencumbered by self-interest and divided loyalties. Doing so in a physician-patient relationship may mean the difference between life and death. Because the physician is the patient's advocate, the patient relies on the physician for professional, objective help.

Boundaries blur easily, however, especially when the patient and doctor feel a strong emotional attachment. When this happens, conflict may arise and the quality of care is often adversely affected.

Below, the authors briefly describe some of the boundary conflicts that can take place in a physician-patient relationship.

Physician-Employee

If the physician is both boss and doctor, numerous problems can occur. As the physician, the doctor is the patient's advocate. But as the boss, the physician is the advocate of his own business. A physician may know that an employee-patient is unable to return to work, yet also wish that he would, because his absence is costing money and causing the office to run less smoothly. A physician may also want to reprimand an employee-patient for poor work, yet also know that the employee is incapable of performing to potential because of a medical problem.

Physicians might use their power as supervisors to convince an employee-patient to do something she did not wish to do, even to do something that they would not advise other patients to do. In addition, when other people in the office learn about an employee's medical problems, they may invade that patient's privacy.

JS once had a conversation with one of her nurses regarding the office medical insurance, which did not cover office visits. JS and the nurse decided it would change their relationship if JS were to see him as a patient. Both would be embarrassed, for example, if JS gave him a physical. To allow her nurse to afford regular examinations, she decided to change to a policy that paid for regular physicals. That way he could afford to see an outside physician and their working relationship would not be damaged.

One of JS's office workers was hospitalized for a severe infection. He still had some memory loss when he decided he wanted to return to work JS required a note from his physician before he could return. If she had been his doctor, she might have let her feelings interfere with this office policy.

The best course of action, the authors feel, is not to accept employees as patients.

Physician-Colleague

When physicians treat colleagues, with whom they interact frequently, they become aware of all their strengths and weaknesses. They may also see their colleagues unclothed, which could make them feel very uncomfortable, even belittled. If physicians avoid this situation by not requiring patient-colleagues to undress, they may not provide the necessary care.

Colleague-patients may also become defensive when asked to provide certain personal information on the patient intake form. They may even withhold information necessary to the proper medical care.

Colleagues may feel insecure or uncomfortable about discussing certain weaknesses. For example, suppose a colleague-doctor reveals he is abusing alcohol or drugs. His doctor must then decide whether she should report the information or try to get the colleague help from a service that must then reveal the problem to licensing agencies. No doctor wants to be in this situation.

Finally, the colleague-patient may want to self-diagnose and that diagnosis may differ from that of the physician. At this point, the physician may need to confront the colleague and suggest that she go somewhere where she can get a more objective point of view.

A physician, whose chief of staff required he see a doctor, once asked JS, his friend, if she would see him as a patient. He did not want JS to examine him completely or to get his lab work done, despite her insistence. He then told the hospital administrator that he had seen JS. Shortly afterward, he collapsed from low potassium.

Apparently, he had a colon polyp that was causing him to lose potassium. The hospital chief of staff then sent him to an outside physician chosen by the hospital. He underwent the needed lab work and physical examination and treatment. An unknown and therefore objective physician will find it much easier to set limits and make sure the physician-colleague followed through with the necessary tests.

When JS was a resident, she saw a woman physician who had just had surgery at the hospital where JS was training, even though it was 50 miles from the hospital where the doctor practised. The doctor attending the woman told JS that he was glad to meet another doctor who felt that doctors should not be treated in their own hospitals. He went on to explain that he had had a pneumothorax treated at the hospital where he practised and was embarrassed when the nurses and doctors with whom he worked cared for him. He realized then that if he needed surgery or other medical care in the future, he would go to a hospital other than his own in order to protect his privacy.

A woman resident told JS that she had delivered her baby at her training hospital because of her insurance policy. She found this very embarrassing, as her male colleagues were in the room with her when she delivered. She said that she would never do that again.

A doctor who is friend of the authors cared for a colleague and good friend, who died in his care. He was devastated by the death of his friend. It is hard when physicians have a patient die. It is worse when the patient is a friend.

In an article on the difficulties of treating physician colleagues, published in the July 14, 2003, *American Medical News*, Damon Adams discussed some guidelines on how to be a good medical patient in these circumstances. For example, the doctor should not provide casual, curbside consults and both parties should clarify financial arrangements ahead of time.

The authors recommend that physicians *not* provide medical care for the doctors or colleagues whom they know or interact with frequently, because in such circumstances physicians cannot be objective. JS does treat physicians and nurses whom she did not know before they became patients. She provides the same explanations that she does to all her patients, because she knows that a doctor may not understand an illness outside his area of expertise or may not be able to think clearly because of the illness. JS knows that doctors need the same care and compassion that all patients require.

Unfortunately, she has noticed that nurse and doctor patients may be the least likely to receive compassion.

When the authors are sick, they try to see physicians with whom they do not work and also go to a hospital where they do not work. They thereby protect their privacy and avoid putting their colleagues in a difficult position.

Physician-Family Member

Doctors may be tempted to treat family members, in part because the family member need not pay for the service and might have asked for help. However, when a doctor treats a family member, the care is often less than adequate. The doctor will find it hard to be objective, especially if the family member has a serious illness. The patient may also be troublesome, refusing to listen or be examined physically, or asking for unnecessary pain medicine

JS recently told a teenaged girl that she would not prescribe birth control pills for her without an examination. The girl was shocked, because a relative had been prescribing the pills without an exam.

An aunt of JS asked her to take her blood pressure during a family visit. Much to the amazement of JS, it was 220/130. She strongly suggested that her aunt talk to her physician about taking blood pressure medication as soon as possible. She refused, saying she did not believe she had high blood pressure. Many years later, she died from a cerebral vascular accident.

When JS was in medical school, a fellow classmate told her that she was angry with her husband, a practising physician, because he refused to treat their children. The husband did not think he could be objective. Only when the classmate became a doctor in a medical clinic did she realize her husband had been right and that such a relationship would bias his medical judgment.

The authors know of a tragic situation in which a doctor prescribed pain medication for his wife while she was dying of cancer. He was so depressed that he also took the medicine himself and became addicted to it.

Any doctor knows that relatives often ask for advice over the phone. A relative of JS asked her to prescribe something for her because she had dizziness. JS explained that she could not treat her over the phone. She thought at the time that her relative might have labyrinthitis. The relative did see a physician and was found to have critical aortic stenosis, which required emergency surgery. It was fortunate that JS did not treat her relative over the phone and insisted that she see another physician.

Doctors are complimented when friends and relatives ask for their advice. However, doctors can avoid a lot of grief if they accept the compliment and then send the person to another physician.

When doctors and relatives cross boundaries that they should not cross, the doctors will find it almost impossible to be objective. One physician may withhold needed treatment in order not to upset a lover or partner or may go into denial if the illness is life threatening. If the lover appears to have a serious infectious disease, such as HIV, the physician may not want to know it and thus avoid doing medically necessary tests. After all, if the lover is positive, the physician might be positive as well. In such a situation, the physician may fear exposure and so deny the lover proper care.

JS knew a gay physician whose partner began to exhibit signs of decreasing health. He was short of breath and had a cough. His physician partner did not think the man was at risk for being HIV positive and did not want him to be tested; he even encouraged him not to be tested. When his lover did become sick, he treated him, ordering all the lab work. Finally, a neutral physician, who was present when an X-ray was taken, determined that the life partner had advanced pneumocystis carinii pneumonia and needed to be hospitalized. If the lover had seen another doctor, someone who was less close to him, he might have been treated sooner.

Another gay physician told the authors that the minute his lover became sick with HIV, he sent him to another doctor. He let his lover choose whom he wanted to see and what treatments to take. He tried not to become involved, unless asked, because he felt he could not be objective. He also felt that his partner would listen to him rather than to his physician and did not want that responsibility. This doctor handled the situation in a wiser way than did the doctor in the previous story.

Physician-Business Partner

Financial ties and entanglements may prevent proper treatment. For example, if a physician is indebted to a patient financially, that physician may be reluctant to charge for the services, considering them part of the debt repayment. If a doctor's business partner falls sick, he may feel obligated to see that doctor, although another physician might suit him better.

A physician, a pulmonary specialist whom JS knew, cared for the person from whom he rented his office. When the patient raised the rent, the physician was so angry that he quit being his doctor. Clearly, the behaviour of both parties was inappropriate.

The authors asked several physicians in their study how they felt about crossing boundaries when it came to providing medical care. Here's a summary of some of their responses:

- I would treat a spouse or family member for routine colds, sore throats, arthritis, etc., but would not treat them in the case of a potentially terminal illness. I believe it is a breach of professional boundaries to treat a close personal friend or relative with a serious illness.   .
- Treating the person is not a breach as long as professional records are kept. However, in a moderate to severe illness, it would be best if the professional was not the primary caregiver.
- When it comes to AIDS, I have often been a significant healthcare provider for friends – close friends. This was difficult for me in some ways but easier in others. If you have an open and honest relationship, then it can work. However, I have always been careful to provide care in a team or partnership role.
- Knowing the healthcare system, a professional or family member can offer options that a person may not know about: a distant professional may not know the client well enough to offer these options. I would stress, however, the close family member should *never* be the sole provider when the diagnosis is poor.

Doctors need to heal themselves. They must be healthy if they are to give the best care to others. They can do this by nourishing their own hope for patients. They can also determine, define, and maintain the boundaries of their professional relationships. Boundaries, which are a significant part of a value system, help physicians protect themselves and help them maintain their emotional and spiritual health. The authors hope more research will be done on this worthy topic, as they have found little so far.

13

Dealing with Guilt, Getting Rid of Shame

Strong people make as many mistakes as weak people. The difference is that strong people admit their mistakes, laugh at them, learn from them. That is how they become strong.

Richard Needham, *The Wit and Wisdom of Richard Needham*, 1977

MISTAKES

Everyone makes mistakes and many mistakes are insignificant. A doctor's mistake, however, can cost a life. Americans tend to sue physicians for errors, both avoidable and unavoidable, in some instances causing them to lose their licences to practise. The American system also sometimes punishes doctors harshly for common complications, even if they made no medical errors. A person dying or experiencing complications and another person not wanting these things to occur can trigger a lawsuit. When doctors suffer unmerited punishments, they may feel a false sense of shame.

While based on science, medicine is also an art. Physicians constantly refine their skills, attempting to incorporate new technologies into their therapeutic techniques. They are constantly learning, constantly growing. Physicians learn from the mistakes they make. In their case, because mistakes can have tragic results, learning often comes at a high cost.

The authors recently had the chance to speak with a Canadian medical student who had a sobering but healthy perspective. She felt that because doctors are thoroughly involved in treating their patients, they will make mistakes from time to time that may result in someone's death. She had accepted that this would happen to her one day. The authors hope that if she does lose a patient because of an error she makes, she is able to remember what she believes now. Knowing her as they do, they think she would be shaken, understand the importance of what happened, and learn from the mistake. Her future patients will be the beneficiaries.

Physicians are involved in the *practice* of medicine, which implies a learning and growing process. They do learn an enormous amount as they continue to practise, both through clinical experience and through medical research. For example, Ryan White died of pneumocystis carinii pneumonia (PCP). If his physician had known at the time that trimethoprim/sulfamethoxazole (Bactrim) could prevent PCP pneumonia, Ryan would have lived longer. Since his death, researchers have discovered how to prevent and treat PCP pneumonia; rarely does a patient die of it today. Current HIV patients benefit from what doctors did not know or understand just ten years ago.

Physicians are fallible. They can miss a diagnosis, give into pressures from Health Maintenance Organizations in the US or by budgetary restraints in other countries not to do "excessive" tests or to refer to an expensive specialist, take the word of a physician in training without double-checking, or make any number of other mistakes that prove how human they really are.

In *Letting Go of Shame*, Ronald and Patricia Potter-Effron (1989) explain that when a person feels he did something wrong and needs to correct that wrong, he is feeling guilt. When a person feels that the mistake he has made proves he is a defective human being and that he is the problem, he is feeling shame. While a guilty person focuses on misdeeds or transgressions, a person filled with shame focuses on personal shortcomings, believing that if he were good enough, he would not have made the mistake.

A guilty person may fear, or even expect, punishment. A person filled with shame may fear rejection or abandonment, believing no one would want someone so flawed and useless.

Shame is toxic, even immobilizing. Guilt, on the other hand, can be a healthy force for correction. Healthy guilt allows people to hold on to self-esteem and address any feelings of guilt that may be present.

In one section of the excellent book *Self-Esteem*, the authors Matthew McKay and Patrick Fanning (1987) focus on common types of mistakes people make. The authors have added their own examples.

- Errors of fact. Examples: writing down the wrong phone number or the wrong dose of an antibiotic

- Failure to reach a goal. Examples: not completing a committee assignment or becoming chief of staff
- Missed opportunities. Example: not marrying someone or not being given the first choice of residencies
- Overindulgence in pleasures. Examples: drinking too much at a party or overspending
- Inappropriate emotional outbursts. Example: yelling at a spouse, children, or staff members
- Violation of a moral code. Example: lying about needing to work late before heading off to a bar.

Readers can ask themselves if they have made mistakes that fit into the above categories, then reframe those errors, putting them into perspective in the following ways:

Mistakes as Teachers

A mistake can teach. If a doctor has an inappropriate emotional outburst, he may begin working on ways to reduce stress or learn meditation or relaxation techniques.

Mistakes as Warnings

Sometimes people don't change until consequences force them to do so. For example, a doctor might have one too many emotional outbursts at work so that a valued staff member quits and two waiting patients decide to seek the services of another physician. She might then realize she must change. This is not the most comfortable way for change to come about but, sadly, it's the way far too many people learn.

Mistakes as a Prerequisite for Spontaneity

If doctors don't act because they fear making a mistake, they will never grow and develop. They have to be willing to learn new treatments, new procedures, and more effective ways of doing things, even if they have to stretch their comfort zone to do so. For example, if a resident is unwilling to put in a central line because she fears she cannot do so correctly, she will never learn the procedure. The resident can request the presence of an experienced physician who will help if a problem arises while learning the technique.

WHAT PHYSICIANS FEAR

Physicians are afraid of some of the following, according to Robert Buckman (1998). They feel:

- Fear of being blamed. If a doctor brings bad news, the patient or family may believe the doctor is at fault. Doctors know little about what to do when the disease has no cure.
- Fear of the untaught. Since there have been few guidelines about treating the dying, doctors might fear being unable to do so properly.
- Fear of eliciting a reaction. A physician may not know how to cope with a patient who cries or becomes very angry during a meeting about a terminal condition.
- Fear of saying 'I don't know.' In clinical practise, fear of showing ignorance stands in the way of developing trust and an honest relationship.
- Fear of expressing emotions. When physicians, quite appropriately, do not show panic or rage when a patient is facing death, the patients may feel their emotional control reveals them to be unfeeling or uncaring. Doctors should not be afraid of their own tears.
- Own fears of illness/death. The physician's own fear of dying may, in extreme circumstances, lead to avoiding any communication with the dying patient.
(Buckman, 1998)

Physicians who believe they have no faults and chide others for the minutest errors place too great a burden on themselves, their staff, and their patients. They should remember that everyone makes mistakes. David Smith, the founder of the Haight/Ashbury Free Clinics in San Francisco, often reminds physicians that "the D in MD does not stand for 'divinity.'"

Physicians strive to master their profession. There's nothing wrong with that, as long as they do not equate mastery with perfection. When doctors make a mistake, they must review their actions to determine what they can learn. Feeling guilty may be healthy unless they begin to obsess about the error.

Shame, however, is never productive. Yet everyone experiences shame from time to time. Everyone has felt that sense of "I'll never amount to anything in this profession." If doctors forget that errors just reveal that they are human and feel instead that their error means they are evil, bad, or worthless, they will lose the confidence that is essential to their proper performance and to their patients' sense of well-being.

When doctors begin to feel shame, they might try several simple exercises. They can:

- Accept the feeling of shame, acknowledging it, breathing with it, and letting it be. While doing so doesn't feel good, resisting the feeling will feel far worse in the end. Everyone knows that attacking a feeling – *any feeling* – and demanding that it go away, never works.
- Work on methods and techniques to decrease and eliminate the distorted thoughts that strengthen shame. The following simple method works for many people. Silently and as often as necessary, they say "let it go" each time a shameful thought surfaces. They make a habit of this approach. Eventually, the shameful thought does not surface as often. As it disappears, they focus on the present moment, saying "PAY ATTENTION TO RIGHT NOW." They need to repeat this over and over until it becomes second nature to react this way.
- Affirm their self-worth, acknowledging their gifts and accomplishments. When they begin to feel shame about something, they can focus on all the times in the past when they received praise for their work. They can recall the times when they felt proud of what they had accomplished. They will begin to find that these positive moments far outweigh the moments when they felt worthless because of a mistake.

Doctors will understand that letting go can involve:

- Accepting self-worth and growing from mistakes
- Recognizing that it was a mistake, rather than denying it
- Acknowledging responsibility for the mistake and the need to make amends when necessary.
- Understanding that a mistake does not define who a person is.

NEUROTIC GUILT VERSUS HEALTHY GUILT

Some people hold on to absolute core beliefs, which they may have learned in early childhood. After doing something wrong, they might say, "I shouldn't make mistakes. Only stupid people do that." Even when such irrational positions are challenged, they continue to generate guilt. This type of guilt is neurotic.

When adults hold childhood beliefs that have become valued ethical or moral rules, they feel conflict and guilt if they break or defy these rules. When this occurs a person can ask some questions:

- Did I intentionally intend to hurt someone else?
- Did I know better at the time? – then, that is, not now.
- Did I ignore information I already had that would have kept me from harming someone else? For example, Did I know I needed to check that patient's chart rather than rely on memory, but didn't because I was tired?

Anyone who responds affirmatively to any of the above questions is probably feeling some healthy guilt.

Neurotic guilt, on the other hand, is based upon unrealistic expectations people place upon themselves. It tends to be fueled by thinking errors such as:

- Expressing shoulds. When a person tells himself that he *should* (ought, must, have to) or *shouldn't* do something, he is defining moral imperatives in absolutist language. He may *prefer* or *wish* he had done something else. If he thinks about it for a while and then lets it go, he is responding in a healthy way. If he obsesses, reminding himself over and over again that he "should have" done something differently (which is, of course, impossible), he can trigger feelings of neurotic guilt.
- Taking excessive responsibility. Scott Peck, author of *The Road Less Traveled* (1986), has a sign on his desk that reminds him when he begins to take on too much responsibility. It reads: "Quit taking care of the world. That's my job. Love, God."

Physicians do not need to feel they are responsible for everyone and everything, trying to exert control over things they cannot control and blaming themselves when anything goes wrong. It's simply a fact that some patients are too sick to be cured – that is nobody's fault.

One way to combat these errors of thought is to question their truth: Are the *shoulds* just a holdover from childhood messages? Are they something picked up in adulthood? Are they reasonable?

Do they consider the complexities of any given situation? Can fallible human beings meet these expectations or are they perfectionist ideals guaranteed to lower self-esteem? Those who ask themselves what they *want* to do rather than what they *should* do will find better answers.

Most of the time doctors are not doing anyone any favours by being over- or hyper-responsible. In the long run this can make people overly dependent upon doctors and lessen their sense of self.

Doctors can detach, feeling genuine compassion for people without becoming enmeshed in their problems. Too often, however, some doctors interpret their feelings of compassion as an obligation to get involved. Many people need, want, and desire help. But doctors cannot do everything. When they begin doing things for patients that the patients could do for themselves, they are sending a message that the patients are not competent. The longer doctors treat patients this way – as if they were children – the more patients will grow to resent such treatment and their doctors.

When physicians find themselves tempted to become too involved or excessively committed, they can ask themselves several simple questions:

• Did the person ask for my help?
• Is the individual doing at least half of the work?
• Am I doing something I can afford to do emotionally? Financially? In terms of time? Physically?

If the answer to any of these questions is negative, it's time for those doctors to back away, particularly if they are beginning to feel resentful.

The steps above may seem simple, but it's amazing how many physicians never try them and regret it later when they are sick, resentful, or burned out. Simple adherence to some simple principles and remembering to ask some basic questions could do away with much of the neurotic guilt felt in life.

There are times when even the most well-meaning people make a mistake or hurt others – and the fault is indeed theirs. Sometimes people behave in an inconsiderate or rude way or forget to do something they promised to do. They can inconvenience someone or hurt their feelings. AC remembers a couple he was counselling who had to travel over 30 miles to their appointment. One evening, having misread his schedule, AC did not show up for the appointment.

When he realized what had happened, he felt guilty for having inconvenienced the couple needlessly.

How do physicians deal with guilt in a healthy way, avoiding any feeling of self-loathing? They may:

- Acknowledge the mistake and the damage done. AC acknowledged to himself that he inconvenienced the couple. He also admitted to the couple that the error was his and said he was sorry that he had wasted their time that evening. While he accepted responsibility, he continued to believe he was a good person who always tried to do his best. When doctors admit they have wronged a patient or family by keeping them waiting or missing an appointment, they are behaving appropriately and with sensitivity. It is not appropriate for doctors to blame others for their mistakes.

  Of course physicians must be careful what they say in certain situations. They may make diagnostic and treatment errors that have tragic results. For example, a physician may miss a cardiac abnormality when reading an EKG tracing with subtle changes. An error may have been a reasonable mistake within standard medical practice and involved no malpractise. Unfortunately, though, if the doctor were to admit the error without consulting an attorney first, he or she might be sued. Physicians are expected to be all-knowing and all-powerful at all times and American society is litigious. This makes admitting even reasonable clinical mistakes a complex issue.

- Consider making amends by apologizing, writing a letter, or making a phone call, if appropriate. Is there some way to correct the wrong done? AC, for example, apologized to the couple for not keeping his appointment and rescheduled them as soon as it was convenient. He then sent them flowers for their trouble.

- Be compassionate with themselves. No one is as smart or insightful or as capable as she would like to be. While doctors are always fallible and never perfect, they can still aim to be the best physicians possible, both clinically and ethically. They can admit to making mistakes, yet still know they are competent and caring. Everything a person does defines them – not one mistake.

- Be accountable. All actions have consequences, so if a price must be paid, it should be paid. For physicians, the consequences may be significant. They may also have to accept consequences they did not foresee. An anesthesiologist whom the authors knew became addicted to several of the drugs he used in his practice. He had self-injected these drugs just before surgeries and carried out his duties while under the influence, putting his patients at great risk. Eventually, superiors found out and told him to get treatment or give up his licence. He decided to go to residential treatment for six months. When he returned to his former hospital to work, he apologized to the staff and to his colleagues. He agreed to random drug testing and to attend Narcotics Anonymous meetings regularly as a condition of his employment. He also spoke to groups of physicians about the dangers of self-medication.

- Learn from the mistake. Those who realize there is something missing in their knowledge, medical skill, or ability to communicate and understand the feelings of others may learn whatever it takes to help them avoid repeating the mistake in the future.
- Ask to be forgiven. The responsibility of the person who made the mistake is to admit the mistake, try and correct the error, and learn from that mistake. There is, of course, no guarantee that if a person apologizes to someone he has wronged that the wronged person will be forgiving. Once the person at fault has made the necessary amends, he can try to forgive himself at some point and can ask his God (or wiser self) to forgive him.

FINDING COMPASSION

Compassion is at the core of self-acceptance; it allows people to accept others and themselves in a complete way. Compassion is a spiritual attribute with three components: understanding, acceptance, and forgiveness.

A young resident, Gail D., was upset that she had not recognized the signs of a ruptured spleen in a patient. What upset her even more than her own failure was that a fellow resident, whom she did not respect, had found them.

Gail's attending physician tried to calm her by saying that it was a very difficult diagnosis because the patient had had no symptoms for ten days. Finally the patient's hemoglobin began to drop and the resident on duty ordered an ultrasound.

Over time, Gail accepted that she had made a mistake. She recognized that her knowledge was limited and that she needed to learn more about the underlying symptoms of this condition. She also realized that she had unfairly judged her fellow resident. She apologized to the patient and the attending physician, neither of whom were upset. She also apologized to her fellow resident for her past "snide" remarks, thereby opening the door for future cooperation, not competition.

SELF-DEFEATING CORE BELIEFS

These beliefs often come down to a simple matter of fantasy versus reality. Those who believe perfection is possible will always experience frustration and defeat because perfection is a fantasy.

Another fantasy is: If I fail at any task, there must be something wrong with me. I must be worthless. The fact is that everyone fails at many tasks in life. It all depends upon how a person defines failure; if someone learns something valuable, then it's not failure. When Thomas Edison was testing possible filament material for the electric light bulb, he was asked how it felt to fail so many times. He remarked, "Fail? Far from it. I now know three thousand things I must not use."

Core beliefs, whether acquired from parents, teachers, society, or by oneself, can and often need to be rewritten. It's possible to change the script if the desire to do so is there. Table 2 lists self-defeating beliefs on the left and the beliefs that may replace them on the right.

Even when beliefs appear valid based upon earlier and often compelling experiences, individuals must critique them until they understand how well the evidence does or does not support those beliefs. An individual should also understand how old beliefs may harm and interfere with well being. A new mature belief, which replaces an old belief, should meet the standards of truth and goodness. Individuals, then, may ask:

- What evidence do I have that a belief is true? More importantly, what evidence do I have that it isn't true? How well does it hold up?
- Is this belief positive? Will holding this belief contribute to my well being? Does it help me achieve my goals? Sometimes the answer is negative. For example, beliefs that lead a person to be suspicious and distrustful are not helpful.

TABLE 2
REPLACING SELF-DEFEATING CORE BELIEFS

Self-Defeating Core Belief	*New Mature Core Belief*
I must be the best.	I have intrinsic value as a person, no matter what I accomplish.
I must not show my emotions.	All feelings are acceptable.
The bad things I've done are unforgivable.	I have the right to forgive myself.
I am ashamed of my past addictions.	I am learning to be sober.
I failed, so I must be a terrible person.	It is okay to make mistakes and learn from this. This is how I grow as a person.
People can't be trusted.	I can learn to trust others selectively.
I should never make mistakes.	It is okay to make mistakes, as long as I am accountable and doing my best.
If people knew me as I really am, they would not like me.	My friends will accept me as I am.
If you can't do it perfectly, don't do it at all.	All I can ask of myself is to do my personal best.
If I am not right all the time, I will not be respected.	I can allow myself to be wrong. I don't need to be perfect to have others like me.
If a patient dies, I am a failure.	I am a competent and hard working doctor, but I can't prevent all patients from dying.

Most people can remember someone who hurt them or was untrustworthy, for many are untrustworthy and hurtful. Still, those people can also remember many people who could be trusted, would pay back a loan, show up for a meeting, and be generous with their time.

The truth is that many people can be trusted with many things. It is also true that no one is perfect and that everyone makes mistakes. No one has a perfect trust record – not even the authors. Even a person who considers herself trustworthy must admit that she has failed others at times. For example a person who can be trusted to respect the feelings of others may have a hard time showing up for appointments on time. That person could be trusted with many important matters but not necessarily with those of lesser importance. Trustworthiness varies greatly, depending upon the person and what you are entrusting them with.

Failing to trust others can be isolating, lead to loneliness, and prevent close friendships and loving relationships from developing. Lack of trust in others can also contribute to depression, chronic anger, and feelings of emptiness. Whatever protection anyone receives by expecting very little from others comes at a high price. AC has had many clients who came to realize that the very wall that protected them from others had become a prison.

If the old belief carries too much negative baggage, replace it with a new core belief that is:

- Affirming
- Flexible, avoiding absolutist language such as "everyone" and "no one"
- Allows growth
- Avoids judgmental words such as "should," "ought," "must," "always," and "never"
- Has been examined critically and is consistent with a wide range of your personal experience.

To shift from the self-defeating to the new and mature is not easy. It can take conscious discipline not to slip back into old patterns of behavior and thinking. However, these new, more mature ways of looking at oneself and the world will become just as ingrained as the old, self-defeating ways were.

New and mature thinking involves forgiving oneself while also accepting responsibility and accountability for mistakes. Readers might want to consider the following meditation, created by the authors, in order not to slip back into perfectionism and irrational self-demands:

> I wish this mistake had not occurred, but I did all I knew to do at the time given the limits of my knowledge and self-awareness. I am learning to accept myself without passing judgment. I do not like what happened, but it does not make me unworthy or useless. I can do nothing to change the past. No matter how unfortunate my decision or action, I still accept myself, take responsibility for my decision and action, and will do my best to move on. I accept that I am like a lot of other people, struggling, often slipping, and surviving as best as I can. I will not continually revisit this mistake; I will continually learn from it. It is over. I can let it go.

Being a physician who takes care of the dying and their families is hard work that makes great emotional and physical demands. Self-care makes it possible to remain healthy and strong when in the midst of so much pain. There will be times when doctors feel guilty over a mistake they made and times when they blame themselves unfairly that a very sick patient died even after they had done everything they knew. At those times doctors need to keep toxic shame from eating away at their self-esteem and self-respect. They also need to recognize that feeling guilty is not evidence that they are guilty. It is easy to feel guilty when expecting too much of oneself.

Compassion for human fallibility opens the heart and helps people become less judgmental of others. It is as important a part of self-care as a healthy diet, regular exercise, avoiding toxic substances, and getting enough sleep. (Chapter 4 gives information about sleep and how to correct problems in this area.)

ALCOHOL AND OTHER DRUGS:
THE DANGEROUS WAY TO REDUCE STRESS

But I do nothing upon myself, and yet I am my own executioner.
John Donne (1572–1632), *Devotions Upon Emergent Occasions and Death's Duel*

First you take a drink, then the drink takes a drink, and then the drink takes you.

F. Scott Fitzgerald (1896–1940)

Day after day doctors experience death and suffering and hurt and often feel helpless to do much about it. Naturally they want and deserve a little relief every now and then. Some may have a few drinks to unwind. Others may be tempted by a jolt of cocaine, a hit off a joint, or the euphoric rush of Fentanyl.

The relief, however, is temporary, very temporary. When the drug wears off, the stress still exists and the only place to go is back to the alcohol or drugs. Doctors certainly know how addictions begin and take over lives. They know that drinkers or addicts come to need more and more alcohol or drugs to decrease stress and that before long their lives are out of control. Knowing is not always enough, though, since some doctors turn to alcohol and drugs for relief anyway.

Max P. was a 50-year-old physician. He had built a successful practice working with HIV patients, although he had not really planned to do so. He was gay and practised medicine in a large city when AIDS first came into public awareness in the early 1980s. Gay patients who were HIV positive sought him out because they knew he would react to them with compassion and understanding. By the 1990s, he had worked with over 800 AIDS and HIV patients, many of whom were his friends. Over the course of nearly ten years he'd seen nearly 300 of his patients die. He was witness to every step of their suffering, including loss of financial security, health, and good looks.

Max P. was unprepared to handle the level of emotional pain he experienced on a daily basis for those ten years. He covered his pain with alcohol, narcotics, and cigarettes. He finally came to the point that he could not handle the stress of running his own practice, so he closed it and became director of a community HIV clinic. One day he had a seizure as a result of taking multiple drugs. Even then he denied that he had a problem.

The state medical board intervened. He lost his licence, but still refused help. At this point, his whereabouts are unknown. The tragedy is that he was an excellent physician who could no longer practice because he denied he had a substance abuse problem.

Robert W. was an intensive care physician who enjoyed the high and the energy he got from stimulants. He once used so many of

TABLE 3

STANDARD DRINKS OF VARIOUS BEVERAGES

Beverage	Amount/oz	Amount/ml
Beer or wine cooler	12	341
Wine	5	142
80 proof distilled spirits	1.5	43

All contain approximately 0.5 ounces of or 17 ml of pure alcohol. Canadian definitions of standard drink are the same as in the US

Source: Canadian Centre on Substance Abuse, 2003

them that he lost consciousness from a cardiac arrhythmia and was admitted to an ICU. He also continued to deny his problem and to use. Eventually his use hurt his work performance. Colleagues eventually sat him down and told him that his memory was becoming impaired. He finally agreed to go to a treatment centre and has become a better physician because of it.

In order for doctors to keep track of how much they are drinking, it helps to know about amounts and tolerances. Table 3 compares different beverages and how much it takes to equal one standard drink (National Institute on Alcohol Abuse and Alcoholism, 2003).

National Institute of Alcohol Abuse and Alcoholism (NIAAA) Recommendations

NIAAA states that moderate alcohol use does not cause problems for most people. Moderate use is defined as one standard drink a day for women and two standard drinks a day for men. While the average number of drinks per week is the usual statistic in population studies, one drink taken each day may not have the same medical or social consequences as drinking seven drinks on one weekend day (Werch, Gorman and Marty, 1987, NIAAA, 1992).

Not everyone can drink, however. Persons who should not drink are:

• Pregnant women
• Recovering alcoholics

- Those under age 21
- Those with medical conditions such as liver disease
- Anyone taking certain medications
- Anyone planning to drive, use heavy machinery, or needing to remain alert to perform certain duties.
  (NIAAA, 2003)

The National Survey on Drug Use and Health published periodically by the Substance Abuse and Mental Health Services Administration (SAMHSA) reported in December 2003 that current drinkers in the US averaged three drinks per day when they drank alcohol. Among current drinkers only, men drank an average of four drinks per day, while women drank an average of two drinks on drinking days. The average number of drink days cited for the previous month varied by sex as well. Men drank on 9.9 days out of the last 30 days, while women drank on only 6.7 days. Overall 51 per cent of Americans had drunk alcohol in the previous 30 days (SAMHSA, 2003).

Other researchers put more importance on the average number of drinks per week. For example when men drink more than fourteen drinks per week and women drink more than seven, they have higher incidences of health problems such as hypertension and cancer, as well as other health problems (NIAAA, 1995).

One Canadian report on the rate of alcohol abuse revealed that the incidence of heavy drinking (usually more than five standard drinks on drinking days) consisted of 8.8 per cent of Canadians in general. When this was broken down by sex, 13.6 per cent of men drink this much when they drink, whereas 4.1 per cent of women do so. Regarding frequency, the number of all Canadians who drink at least once a week stood at 34.9 per cent (Northwest Territories Bureau of Statistics, 1996).

Family Risk Measure

Another way to assess alcohol problems, included in the Project MATCH Assessment Feedback protocol, is to determine family risk. Points for each relative who is positive for drug/alcohol problems are as follows:

- If father is positive add two points
- If mother is positive add two points

- For each brother who is positive add two points
- For each sister who is positive add two points
- For each grandparent who is positive add one point
- For each uncle or aunt who is positive add one point

A person with a score of

- 0–1 is at a low risk
- 2–3 points is at medium risk
- 4–6 is at high risk
- 7 and above is at very high risk

of developing alcohol problems. (Miller, 1995)

The CAGE

The CAGE is a rapid screening questionnaire used successfully to identify a high likelihood of alcoholism.

C   Have you ever felt you ought to Cut down on your drinking?
A   Have people Annoyed you by criticizing your drinking?
G   Have you ever felt bad or Guilty about your drinking?
E   Have you ever had a drink in the morning (Eye opener) to steady your nerves or get rid of a hangover?

Each positive answer is worth one point. Those who respond positively to two or more of the questions are very likely to be alcoholics (Bradley et al., 1998).

Tolerance

Social drinkers usually feel the effects of alcohol after one or two drinks. This serves as an "early warning system" to let them know that things could get out of control if they consume any more. When those with a high tolerance for alcohol drink, they may be able to consume fairly sizable quantities without feeling much in the way of warnings or negative effects. This can be very dangerous because the apparent tolerance masks the very real physical damage to the brain and other organs that is taking place. These drinkers resemble those who cannot feel pain and have been accidentally injured.

A person's peak Blood Alcohol Concentration (BAC) level during a typical drinking week reflects his or her level of tolerance for alcohol. Some people reach higher than normal BAC levels without feeling the normal effects social drinkers experience. A higher tolerance, although partly hereditary, may be a serious sign that alcohol problems are present or are likely to develop.

If a person can drink more than one or two drinks in an hour and still feel little effect, he may be developing a problem with tolerance. Women are more sensitive than men to the effects of alcohol.

Alcohol Use Disorders Identification Test (AUDIT)

The World Health Organization uses the AUDIT in many countries in order to identify persons who may have alcohol problems and need further physical and laboratory evaluation by a physician (Balor, 1989, Miller, 1995). (See Table 4)

After answering the questions, add up the numbers attached to each answer to obtain the total record score. The following scores indicate the severity of the alcohol problem:

- 0–7: low
- 8–15: medium
- 16–25: high
- 26–40: very high

Other Drugs

The following levels of risk were used in the Project MATCH Study to determine the greater risk for negative consequences among alcohol abusers who also use drugs as opposed to alcohol abusers who do not. Doctors may ask which level of risk they think applies to them (Miller, 1995).

HIGH RISK FOR SERIOUS CONSEQUENCES:
Any use of cocaine or crack, or any use of heroin, methadone, or other opiates, or frequent use (more than three months of at least one use a week) of any other drug class except tobacco, including:

- marijuana, hash, THC
- amphetamines, stimulants, diet pills

TABLE 4

THE AUDIT QUESTIONNAIRE

Circle the number that describes best your drinking pattern:

1) How often do you have a drink containing alcohol?
   0=Never   2=2–4 times a month   4=4+ times a week
   1=Monthly   3=2–3 times a week.

2) How many drinks containing alcohol do you have on a typical day
   when you are drinking?
   0=One or two   2=Five or six   4=Ten or more
   1=Three or four   3=Seven to nine

3) How often do you have six or more drinks on one occasion?
   0=Never   2=Monthly   4=Daily or almost daily
   1=Less than monthly 3=Weekly

4) How often during the last year have you found that you were not
   able to stop drinking once you started?
   0=Never   2=Monthly   4=Daily or almost daily
   1=Less than monthly 3=Weekly

5) How often during the last year have you failed to do what was
   normally expected from you because of drinking?
   0=Never   2=Monthly   4=Daily or almost daily
   1=Less than monthly 3=Weekly

6) How often during the last year have you needed a first drink in the
   morning to get yourself going after a heavy drinking session?
   0=Never   2=Monthly   4=Daily or almost daily
   1=Less than monthly 3=Weekly

7) How often during the last year have you had a feeling of guilt or
   remorse after drinking?
   0=Never   2=Monthly   4=Daily or almost daily
   1=Less than monthly 3=Weekly

8) How often during the last year have you been unable to remember what
   happened the night before because you had been drinking?
   0=Never   2=Monthly   4=Daily or almost daily
   1=Less than monthly 3=Weekly

TABLE 4/continued

---

9) Have you or someone else been injured as a result of your drinking?
    0=No   2=Yes, but not in last year   4=Yes, during the last year

10) Has a relative or friend or a doctor or other health worker been
    concerned about your drinking or suggested you cut down?
    0=No   2=Yes, but not in last year   4=Yes, during the last year

After answering the questions, add up the numbers attached to each answer
to obtain the total score.

In determining response categories it has been assumed that one drink contains 10g of alcohol (Balor, 1989).

- tranquilizers
- barbiturates

MEDIUM RISK FOR SERIOUS CONSEQUENCES:
Any lifetime nonprescription use but not frequent use of (i.e., three
months or less of weekly use) of any drug class, except for tobacco,
opiates, or cocaine, but including:

- marijuana
- amphetamines, stimulants, diet pills
- tranquilizers
- barbiturates

LOW RISK FOR SERIOUS CONSEQUENCES:
No use of above drugs, although may use tobacco

Alcohol is not harmful when used in moderation. It becomes a
problem when its consumption begins to cause mental or physical
damage resulting from addiction. Physicians need to be very aware of
this, since the abuse of alcohol and other drugs may put them in situations in which they make an impaired and costly medical decision.

Serum Chemistry

The following blood tests can become elevated with excessive drinking and are an indicator of the degree of physical damage caused by alcohol. Sometimes, however, heavy drinkers may register normal levels:

- SGOT/SGPT
- GGTP
- Bilirubin (total)
- Uric acid

Serum chemistry often speaks the truth when patients will not, although elevations might be due to other disorders. A young physician entered the hospital with recurring pancreatitis. He denied drinking but his GGTP was elevated. When presented with the blood work results, he admitted to heavy drinking. He was referred to a treatment centre.

Self-Administering Controlled Substances

Doctors who write prescriptions for themselves or medicate themselves with controlled substances have a serious problem. Doing so may lead to continued use and unethical behaviour.

What To Do

Following are some courses of action for those who may have a problem with alcohol or other drugs, as indicated by one of the above screening tests. They can:

- Attempt to cut down consumption of alcohol to recommended limits and find alternatives to deal with the stress that comes with treating dying patients. Most moderation management drinking groups suggest that you go through 30 days of sobriety before resuming drinking at recommended levels. With severe problems, however, abstinence will be necessary, if not lifesaving.
- Seek the support of Alcoholics Anonymous (AA) or Narcotic Anonymous (NA) groups. Anonymity is the foundation of these groups, so there is no need to worry that your problem will be exposed or become the object of judgment and speculation. AA

and NA groups meet in nearly every city and town; it's easy to call for assistance, as all city directories list AA numbers. Groups outside of your own area make it easier to protect your anonymity.

- Ask a physician/addictionologist or a psychologist specializing in substance abuse to do an evaluation to see if there is a problem with alcohol or other drugs.
- Ask a physician/addictionologist about medicines that help reduce craving, if an evaluation indicates a problem that either temporary or permanent abstinence would help
- Consider that an orderly regimen of detoxification may be necessary if they experience withdrawal symptoms.
- Ask themselves whether they might have a psychiatric disorder and, if so, seriously consider seeking treatment for the problem in order to achieve quality sobriety. Chemical dependency is often associated with an underlying psychiatric disorder such as depression or anxiety. There are inpatient programs that specialize in treating physicians, so doctors can ask the professionals they contact to help them decide whether such a program is appropriate.

Physician impairment was defined in 1973 by the American Medical Association Council on Mental Health as "the inability to practice medicine by reason of physical or mental illness, including alcoholism or drug dependence" (AMA Council on Mental Health, 1973). In 1991, JAMA conducted an extensive study: "Resident Physician Substance Use in the US." This study found that medical students and residents used fewer illegal drugs than others of similar age in the general population. However, they found that this same group used more alcohol and benzodiazepines. Practicing physicians used even more benzodiazepines and minor opioids. The more frequently they prescribed these to their patients or the greater the accessibility to these drugs, the more they used them. The prevalence of chemical dependency among physicians in this and some other studies was in the 10 to 15 per cent range (Hughes, et al., 1991).

Substance abuse and substance dependence make up the two major categories of substance-related disorders in the DSM-IV-TR of the American Psychiatric Association. Substance abuse, the lesser diagnosis, is defined as a "maladaptive use leading to significant impairment or distress," with one or more of these features:

- Failure to fulfill major role obligations

- Use of the substance in which there is physical damage to oneself, or in which the result is physical damage to property (e.g., a car wreck)
- Legal problems, such as arrest for disorderly conduct or driving while intoxicated (DWI) related to substance abuse
- Persistent or frequent interpersonal problems related to intoxication, such as outbursts with a spouse or with colleagues at work.

Substance dependence involves such symptoms as tolerance, withdrawal, using larger amounts than intended, and continued use despite adverse physical or psychological consequences (Task Force on DSM-IV, 2000).

Alcoholism refers to either abuse or dependency as defined above. To the surprise of some, many alcoholics are not addicted to alcohol, drink beer only, don't have to drink every day, do the majority of their drinking on weekends, have families, and go to work every day. Yet they are alcohol abusers nonetheless. One day they may become alcohol dependent as well.

A retired physician who came to see AC worried that he had developed alcohol problems over the year following a traumatic experience at a medical centre, which resulted in the loss of his job. AC found no evidence of dependency or need for detoxification. It was clear, however, that the physician was drinking excessively and was experiencing hangovers and occasional blackouts. Due to his high motivation, he stopped drinking on his own, came in for outpatient counselling for several months, and attended AA regularly. Several months after coming in, he reported that he was sober and was enjoying his retirement with his wife, gardening, and his grandchildren.

Some may drink beer or use alprazolam or hydrocodone/acetaminophen, because doing so makes them feel good – or at least less stressed. No problem may exist at first, but for some use may gradually escalate over time. This increased use may be partly in reaction to stressful situations, such as financial problems, marital problems, or chronic pain. Because many people drink a lot, such drinking may even seem normal

After a while, some find that they are continuing to drink or use drugs even though doing so is hurting them or causing harm to others. They are unable to see that they are unhappy because of the alcohol or drugs. While they are troubled, the alcohol or drugs appear to help, lifting spirits and reducing discomfort, at least for a while. These people tend to blame others for their inability to function well at work, marital problems, excessive sensitivity to criticism, increased anger, memory problems, or decreased self-confidence. They begin to make excuses for their substance abuse, saying "I only drink on weekends," or "I can quit any time," or "I only drink beer," or "Nobody is going to find out," or "At least I don't drink like Jack does."

This defensiveness, which involves blaming or feeling out of touch with one's feelings, is characteristic of denial. Denial allows substance abusers to continue to get worse, without working on their problem.

Donald Goodwin, in an article published in 1992 titled "Alcohol: Clinical Aspects," states that alcoholism does not necessarily follow a certain sequence. Not all alcoholics lose control as soon as they begin drinking or cannot stop until their health and finances deteriorate terribly. Some heavy drinkers, according to Goodwin, drink moderately for a long period of time and then their drinking begins once again to interfere with their health or their social life (Goodwin, 1989).

Depending on alcohol and other drugs is a very destructive way to cope with the stress of treating dying patients. If doctors think alcohol or addictive prescription drugs have become a significant part of their life, they might take some time to sit and meditate about where they think the abuse of chemicals might take them. They can play out a scenario in their mind – all the way to the end. Is the picture they see a pleasant one? They might also talk with a close friend or a colleague who is not afraid to speak honestly. There is certainly plenty of help out there if they feel they need it. A physician/addictionologist or a psychologist who specializes in addictions can help evaluate the problem and the necessary treatment. Sometimes an inpatient facility is the best choice, in particular a facility that specializes in the treatment of physicians with substance abuse problems.

Identifying and Treating Clinical Depression and Anxiety

Geeze, if I could get through to you, kiddo, that depression is not sobbing and crying and giving vent, it is plain and simple reduction of feeling.

Judith Guest, *Ordinary People*, 1976.

John A. was referred to a hospital committee because his behavior was erratic and he appeared to have a drug problem. He didn't.

However, he did suffer severe anxiety and depression. He had been married several times. To pay his alimony, he had to work at three jobs. He was so exhausted that one day he collapsed at work. Eventually a counsellor helped him to recognize his emotional and physical limits. As a result, he worked out a more equitable alimony payment and was able to quit one of his full-time jobs. He also began an exercise program and lost weight. John had felt that he was a bad person because he had failed at so many marriages. A counsellor helped him begin to work through his guilt and a psychiatrist prescribed antidepressants.

Physicians are not immune to clinical depression, which is a devastating illness that can have serious consequences on a medical practise if not diagnosed and treated. For a doctor to make an informed opinion about whether he or a colleague has clinical depression and might benefit from professional intervention and treatment, he can ask himself whether several of the following have been going on for several weeks most of the time. If the doctor has been feeling:

- Sad
- Guilty
- Low self-esteem
- Irritable and bad tempered
- Suicidal or wishing to die, even with no intent

or experiencing changes in:

- Appetite
- Sleep patterns

or losing:

- Interest in activities and friends
- Hope for the future
- Motivation

he or she might consult the Task Force on DSM-IV, 2000, American Psychiatric Association: Diagnostic and Statistical Manual of Mental Disorders, DSM-IV-TR for formal diagnostic criteria.

Doctors have problems accepting the patient role, according to psychiatrist Michael a'Brook (1990), and are likely to avoid seeking treatment. Doctors are also likely to stop treatment prematurely, even when their psychiatrists are well trained. a'Brook also suspected that much depression among doctors is masked by drug and alcohol abuse.

Several studies over the last 15 years have described the rates of depression and stress among physicians in numerous countries, including the US, England, Sweden, Finland, and Australia. Although the findings are somewhat contradictory and the rates of impairment vary with the measure of stress and depression and the medical disciplines studied, most studies found significant levels of stress, depression, and exhaustion. Still, job satisfaction was generally high. Some studies, for example, reported elevated levels of depression among 20 to 25 per cent of residents in a variety of specialties (Hsu and Marshall, 1987, Reuben, 1989, Hurwitz et al., 1987). Other studies reported moderate levels of depression but high levels of emotional exhaustion and stress (Chambers and Belcher, 1994, Lloyd et al., 1994).

Female doctors appear to be at greater risk than male doctors. Carol North and Jo-Ellyn Ryall (1997) reported that while the suicide rate of male physicians matches that of white men in general in the US population, the suicide rate of women physicians was triple or quadruple the corresponding rate of white women in the US (Council on Scientific Affairs, 1987). Similarly, a 1999 Swedish study asked a random sample of 1,004 general practitioners to participate in a health survey (Sundquist and Johansson, 1999). They found that female general practitioners had a higher risk of impaired health status than male general practitioners. Women physicians also showed significantly greater rates of anxious and depressed feelings than women in the general population. High suicide rates have also been reported for female physicians in studies in Denmark (Arnetz et al., 1987) and Finland (Lindeman et al., 1997).

Physicians, in other studies, have shown overall higher suicide mortality than other professionals (British Medical Association, 1993, Lindeman et al., 1996); women physicians seem to be at even greater risk. Women physicians may be experiencing stress, which leads to depression, while making career decisions in a demanding profession. This stress may then affect their ability to meet the demands of their families at home (Sundquist and Johansson, 1999).

Both male and female physicians have to confront a dark side of medicine in their work, which is not very glamorous. Pediatric ICU fellows, for example, may save the life of a child and then, perhaps an hour later, another child may be on the verge of dying. Jellinek and others (1993) reported in a study that feelings of guilt, fear, worry, sadness, and anger are common, as the pediatric intensive care fellows encounter highly stressed parents and very sick children at great risk of death. Those authors noted that a mistake could make a physician feel like a worthless failure, who has let everyone down. When decisions are to be made to stop treatment or when a family responds to the death of a child, the fellows do not know how much to empathize and how much to detach. If they block their feelings of sadness and disappointment, they risk shutting off their feelings. They will then have trouble turning them on again when they are at home with their own loved ones. If they become too involved, on the other hand, they risk becoming paralyzed with fear and grief. Memories of their own personal losses from divorces or family deaths can also combine with the present crises, bringing on feelings of grief and possibly depression. The authors also wrote that these fellows, who have difficulty accepting their own fallibility, might expect to be free from error and able to stop the death they see all around them. Nurses and others in the ICU share this situation, which is hard for anyone to handle well.

Authors recommended some solutions to program directors, including scheduling regular small group discussions to allow staff to ventilate their feelings about these pressures and providing experienced and supportive mentors to actively help fellows find ways to cope with the impossible expectations.

Fellows and the many residents and physicians who treat seriously ill patients are at risk of using alcohol and self-prescribed drugs when they feel depressed and overwhelmed. If they are feeling depressed and are drinking or using medications in order to cope, they need to stop and get help immediately.

What to Do about Depression

If several of the symptoms on the list above have persisted for several weeks or more in an intense way, or if a person has even thought in a passing manner about taking his or her own life, that person needs to talk to a trusted colleague or friend or place themself under a mental health professional's care and get help immediately. Clinical depression is treatable; it is not something anyone wants to leave untreated for very long.

When deciding to seek therapy, doctors should find a professional who holds a doctoral degree, is licenced, and understands the nature and the stages of grief. Much depression can be traced to grief in one form or another.

Medicals professionals usually see a psychiatrist or psychologist in such situations. Some may prefer to seek a psychotherapy alone (without medication) if:

- No psychosis is present
- Psychotherapy has worked well in the past
- Contraindications to using antidepressants may rule them out
- Antidepressants are unacceptable
- Symptoms of depression are mild to moderate in severity.
(Pradko and Rush, 1999)

Cognitive-behavioral therapy, in particular, has been shown to be of comparable efficacy to antidepressant medications in both the acute and maintenance phases (Blackburn and Moore, 1997). This therapy, which focuses on changing negative thinking patterns and behaviors, is very helpful in most instances. A systematic review of 48 randomized controlled trials of mainly outpatients with mild to moderate depression concluded that 79 per cent of patients receiving no treatment had more symptoms of depression than patients receiving cognitive therapy (Gloaguen et al., 1998, Geddes et al., 2003).

Other psychological treatments have been studied with encouraging results (Geddes et al., 2003). Large randomized controlled trials of adults with mild to moderate depression concluded that interpersonal psychotherapy or problem solving treatment helped improve symptoms of depression in comparison to no treatment, at least in the short term. There were no significant differences between these psychological therapy treatments and the antidepressant drug groups (Elkin et al., 1989, Mynors-Wallis et al., 1995). Unfortunately, neither of these psychological treatments is widely available.

Talk therapy may work very well for some doctors. However, if others find that after several weeks of talk therapy their mood is still the same or has intensified, they may need antidepressant medication to supplement the work they are doing. Combining psychotherapy and medication makes good sense if a person:

- Is suffering a depression so severe that he is unable to function

- Has a history of mood swings that include a manic episode
- Has hallucinations, such as hearing her name being called
- Cannot concentrate during psychotherapy sessions or progress in any way because of the depression
- Has a chronic or recurrent depression, with an incomplete recovery between episodes.

(Burns, 1989, Pradko and Rush, 1999)

Antidepressant medication and psychotherapy usually work best in tandem (Blackburn et al., 1981). A randomized study on depression followed 40 patients who had responded successfully to medication for recurrent major depression, assigning them to one of two groups: routine clinical management or cognitive-behavioral therapy. Antidepressants were discontinued in both groups after 20 weeks. At a two-year follow-up, the two groups differed markedly. Eighty per cent of the clinical management group had relapsed whereas only 25 per cent of the cognitive-behavioral group had had a recurrence of depression (Fava and Rafanelli, 1998). A similar finding involved a meta-analysis of 20 years of studies on panic disorder. Whereas both cognitive-behavioral therapy and medication worked equally well, the results were longer lasting for the cognitive-behavioral group (Clay, 2000).

In any case, doctors should not try to diagnose and prescribe antidepressants for themselves. Depression can create confusion and limit objectivity, so doctors are advised not to treat depression on their own.

IDENTIFYING AND TREATING CLINICAL ANXIETY

When JS was a resident, she was asked to supervise an intern who had been hospitalized for anxiety. This young man, an excellent physician, had been previously assigned to a resident who gave his interns a great deal of freedom and little supervision. The intern panicked and required psychiatric hospitalization. He was later told that he did not have to learn without supervision and was assigned to JS after he was released from the hospital. Perhaps if he had talked about his anxiety earlier, his hospitalization could have been prevented.

In order to decide whether or not one is clinically anxious, a person may consider the following as it relates to the last several months. A person may be clinically anxious who has been feeling:

- Nervous or afraid
- Tense, on edge
- Dizzy
- Irritable, bad tempered
- Afraid that something bad will happen
- Easily tired
- Frequently worried about many things

or has:

- Trouble falling asleep
- Racing or pounding heart
- Been trembling or shaking
- Headaches, neck, or back pain
- Stomach discomfort
- Trouble concentrating
- Racing thoughts
- Been startling easily

See the Task Force on DSM-IV, 2000, American Psychiatric Association: Diagnostic and Statistical Manual of Mental Disorders, DSM-IV-TR for formal diagnostic criteria.

Part Four of this book may help doctors find ways to manage anxiety so that it is no longer troublesome. However, if anxiety symptoms don't seem to be responding to a self-help program or if the anxiety interferes with functioning in a significant way, doctors ought to seek professional assistance.

Cognitive-behavioral psychotherapy can help a person reduce anxiety by providing stress management skills and ways to change the irrational thinking that drives anxiety.

Doctors may also benefit from anxiety lowering medications such as SSRIs, other antidepressants, or buspirone. Unlike the anxiolytics, which are best used on a short-term basis in most cases, these medicines are not addictive or likely to worsen a co-existing depression.

Self-medication is not advisable. Psychiatrists should make such decisions.

14

Problems in Coping

WHEN SLEEP WON'T COME

Sleep is when all the unsorted stuff comes flying out as from a dustbin upset in a high wind.

William Golding, *Pincher Martin: The Two Deaths of Christopher Martin*, 1956

Dealing with death on a day-in, day-out basis, caring for gravely ill patients, and responding to the concerns of family members are all highly stressful and emotionally draining. Physicians need to be rested and alert when these situations arise. This is much easier written than done. The authors know many health professionals, including themselves sometimes, who suffer from bouts of insomnia. Sometimes these professionals are able to turn off the stress of the day. At other times the stress is too great and they simply cannot do so. They toss and turn, fretting over decisions they made during the day and questioning their ability and themselves. They might ask: Could I have handled things differently? What did I miss? Did I do the best I could for that patient this morning? (Or yesterday, or last week, or last year?)

The inability to sleep is common in the medical profession. Up to 50 per cent of the general US population occasionally have problems sleeping and 10 per cent report frequent problems with sleep (Johnson, 1999). Many doctors who routinely care for terminally ill patients manage to hold things pretty well together during the day because they are so busy. At night, though, they find it much harder to let the tensions of the day disappear.

How much sleep a person needs varies. While most people need seven to eight hours, some feel fine with five or six, while some need as many as ten. The basic rule is that if a person feels energetic during the daytime, that person is getting enough sleep.

Insomnia is generally defined as unsatisfying sleep as a result of the following, either alone or in combination.

- Trouble falling asleep
- Waking often in the middle of the night with problems returning to sleep
- Waking one or more hours early and being unable to return to sleep
- Sleep that is not refreshing and not restorative.
  (National Heart, Lung, and Blood Institute, 1995)

Insomnia can be an acute or transient phenomenon, which may or may not be repeated periodically, or it can be a chronic problem that goes on and on. Examples of transient problems include anxiety experienced at tax time, jet lag, time-limited work pressures such as preparing for a hospital accreditation review, and environmental noise. The problems usually last from a few nights to a few weeks. Chronic insomnia, in contrast, occurs on most nights for a month or longer. The causes can be many. They include:

1 Psychiatric problems, such as clinical depression and anxiety disorders
2 Medical causes, such as allergies, chronic pain, hyperthyroidism, or reactions to medications such as steroids, decongestants, or beta-blockers, as well as specific sleep disorders such as sleep apnea and restless legs syndrome
3 Lifestyle choices, which may involve stress on the job, poor exercise habits, the consumption of caffeine after lunch, or other diet deficiencies and excesses
4 Poor sleep habits, such as going to bed at a different time each evening or trying too hard to fall asleep.
   (Hauri and Linde, 1990)

Treatments for insomnia can be either pharmacological or behavioural. Transient insomnia may not require any treatment since the problem usually goes away on its own. However, when impaired performance results from the lack of sleep, short-term use of hypnotics that are short acting and have minimal residual sedation on the next day may be appropriate in many instances.

Medications are less useful when the problem is chronic, although that is controversial. Behavioural techniques are more likely to be effective over the long term (National Heart, Lung, and Blood Institute, 1995). Sedating medications may also be a problem for physicians who may need to function and be alert during the sleep period as a result of on-call duties (Simon, 2000).

Behavioural techniques have been shown to bring about reliable and lasting benefits for persons with insomnia when taught by a mental health professional (Morin et al., 1994, Roth, 2000, Bootzin and Perlis, 1992, Morin and Azrin, 1987, Murtagh and Greenwood, 1995). These strategies include sleep hygiene training, sleep restriction therapy, stimulus control, relaxation therapy, and paradoxical intention. Although several weeks of training may be necessary to see results and effort and persistence are involved, benefits tend to be sustained for months or years (Simon, 2000).

Good sleep hygiene is a set of practices that promote regular and sound sleep. Although insufficient by itself as a treatment for insomnia, it serves as the cornerstone of treatment for insomnia and is recommended first. It consists of the following:

- Waking up at the same time each day (to create a stable circadian rhythm)
- Avoiding all napping
- Going to bed only when sleepy
- Avoiding caffeine four to six hours before bedtime and reducing total daily use
- Avoiding nicotine, which has stimulating properties, for at least four hours before bedtime
- Avoiding using alcohol to bring about sleep, as alcohol is disruptive to good quality sleep
- Eating a light snack at bedtime may help, but a heavy meal will likely interfere with sleep
- Arranging for maximum bright light exposure during waking hours and for maximum darkness and quiet during the desired sleep hours (to strengthen stable circadian rhythm)
- Developing a daily exercise pattern that is completed three to four hours before going to sleep. Low to moderate exercise helps to increase slow-wave sleep, which is the most restful and rejuvenating.
- Developing a bedtime wind-down ritual such as journal-writing about one's feeling and worries for 15 or 20 minutes about an

hour before bedtime, followed by 30 to 45 minutes of relaxing activities such as light reading, watching unexciting television, listening to soft instrumental music or relaxation tapes, taking a warm bath, or meditating.
- Making sure the mattress is comfortable, with adequate neck and back support.
(Simon, 2000, Walsh et al, 1998)

Other behavioural techniques that have proven successful include:

- Relaxation therapies. Progressive muscle relaxation, autogenic training, and abdominal breathing are equally effective in reducing somatic arousal while meditation and imagery reduce cognitive arousal (Hauri, 1981, Simon, 2000)
- Sleep Restriction Therapy. This consists of systematically cutting down the amount of time spent in bed to increase the percentage of time asleep. A person who sleeps an average of five hours per night may be spending seven or eight hours in bed each night. The problem sleeper discovers this by keeping a sleep diary for two weeks in which she records the time spent in bed each night, along with her estimated sleep time. Initially, in this case, the problem sleeper limits the time in bed to five hours. Then every five days, 15 to 30 minutes per night adjustments are made to the bedtime hour, while waking time remains fixed. Time in bed is never reduced below five hours, particularly in the case of the elderly. Since naps are not allowed, the problem sleeper will become temporarily sleepier during the day, until sleep at night approaches the desired duration at a high level of efficiency (Simon, 2000, Walsh et al, 1998).
- Stimulus Control Therapy. Based on conditioning therapy, this therapy involves:
  - Going to bed when sleepy
  - Using the bedroom only for sex and sleep and not for eating, reading, or watching television in order to break the association between bed and activity
  - After about 20 minutes of not sleeping, getting up and going to another room until sufficiently sleepy to try again. In the other room, engaging in activities that are not stimulating, such as reading or watching television but not Internet surfing. This is repeated as often as necessary until the person falls asleep.

- Rising at a regular time in the morning, regardless of time spent asleep
- Not napping during the day

Clinical trials, such as a study by Espie et al. (1989) have documented the efficacy of this approach (Hauri and Linde, 1990).

- Paradoxical Intention. In this less well-known method, the problem sleeper is asked to lie in bed and fight sleep. Since fear of staying awake may inhibit sleep, genuinely attempting to stay awake can prevent performance anxiety (Murtach and Greenwood, 1995, Ascher and Turner, 1979).

Physicians cannot escape the frustration and stress of their work. Each day brings new and often unexpected situations and crises with which they must deal. They do have a choice, however, as to whether or not the stress of their days will stretch over into their nights. By putting into practise some of the very basic things described above, doctors may be more rested, which in the long run will make them more efficient and better able to handle the tension of each day.

It's possible, though, that none of the above may help. There are many sleeping and waking problems or disorders that interfere with sleep, so much so that they harm quality of life and personal health. The suggestions made above will not eliminate these problems, which require some medical treatment.

Some sleep disorders, such as sleep apnea, may even lead to serious illness or endanger public safety because they may cause traffic accidents and work errors. Other disorders include circadian rhythm disorders, limb movement disorder (PLMD), and restless leg syndrome. Certainly anyone who has trouble sleeping and has sinus infections, hypertension, hyperthyroidism, or arthritis should seek treatment. The many causes of sleep disorder include chronic obstructive lung disease, heart disease, gastrointestinal reflux disease, chronic sinusitis, depression, clinical anxiety, and asthma.

Because quality sleep is necessary for mental and physical restoration, those who are unable to sleep well after following the above suggestions or believe they may have a sleep disorder will benefit by asking an internist or family practice doctor for a general history and physical to evaluate treatable medical disorders. Another option would be to go to a sleep disorder centre, which provides diagnostic services and treatment to patients who present with symptoms or features that suggest the presence of a sleep disorder.

Useful information about sleep disorders can be obtained by contacting the American and Canadian organizations listed under Sleep Disorders in the Resources section at the end of this book.

PART FOUR

Reducing Stress

15

Relaxation, Meditation, and Visualization

I made some studies, and reality is the leading cause of stress among those in touch with it. I can take it in small doses, but as a lifestyle, I found it too confining.

Jane Wagner

Adopting the right attitude can convert a negative stress into a positive one.

Hans Selye

Many people bury their anxiety; they pretend it will go away or sooth the tension with alcohol or other drugs. These behaviors will only work for a short term, if at all. There are safe and natural alternatives that can help people reduce their general level of anxiety and muscle tension, tension caused by a particular life situation, and anxiety and tension that interfere with healthy sleep patterns.

RELAXATION SKILLS

Scanning for Tension Points

Scanning is an orderly and effective way to pay attention to the pressure and tension points throughout the body. Scanning will reveal that certain areas of the body, such as the neck and shoulders, store a lot of tension and tightness. On discovering tension at a certain point in the body, a person can take a deep breath and say, "Relax, let it go," while breathing out. To perform a simple body scan, a person can:

- Pay attention to the feet and legs. Notice any tension in toes, feet, and calves. Take a deep breath. Relax.
- Move up the body. Notice any discomfort in the lower back, hips, pelvis, and buttocks. Take a deep breath. Relax.
- Focus on any tension in the diaphragm and stomach. Breathe in and out slowly and deeply for several breaths. Relax.
- Notice any tension in the lungs and chest. Breathe deeply. Relax.
- Move on to the shoulders, neck, and throat. Shrug the shoulders. Roll the head around a few times and then roll it the other way. Notice any tension. Relax.
- Continue on to the forehead, eyes, jaw, and teeth. Notice any tension or pain there. Breathe deeply. Relax.

Deep Abdominal Breathing

Do this exercise in a private place of the home with no interruptions from TV, radio, telephone (unplug it), beeper, or family, once or twice a day for about 5 or 10 minutes. After one or two weeks, increase the time to 15 to 20 minutes a session. To do the exercise,

1 Lie down or sit up in a comfortable chair. Keep your back straight.
2 Scan your body for tension.
3 Put your hand on your abdomen.
4 Breathe in slowly and deeply through your nose and let your belly begin to inflate a little, like a balloon, keeping the abdominal muscles relaxed. Be careful not to breathe too deeply at first, as you might feel dizzy from the oxygen intake.
5 Let your abdomen fall again, while exhaling through your mouth. Continue to take slow, deep breaths that let your relaxed abdomen inflate and deflate.
6 Scan your body again for tension, paying attention to whether the tension decreases. Once skilled at breathing away tension, repeat throughout the day for a minute or two, whether waiting for a phone call or an elevator.

Progressive Muscle Relaxation

This relaxation technique involves tensing individual muscle groups throughout the body and holding the tension for 5 to 10 seconds in order to fatigue the muscles. Notice what the tension feels like. While releasing the tension slowly, say "relax." Finally, notice the sensations that accompany relaxation: warmth, heaviness, and pleasure for about 15 or 20 seconds. It is very important *not* to rush the sequence of tensing and releasing. To do the exercise, you will:

1 Sit in a comfortable position sitting in a quiet room in which you won't be interrupted, with TV and radio off.
2 Clench your right fist tighter and tighter. Hold the tension for about 10 seconds. Relax for about 20 seconds.
3 Clench your left fist. Hold the tension. Relax.
4 Bend your elbows and tense your biceps. Hold the tension. Relax.
5 Wrinkle your forehead by lifting your eyebrows. Hold the tension. Relax and smooth out your forehead.
6 Close your eyes tighter and tighter. Hold the tension. Relax.
7 Clench your jaw. Bite down hard. Hold the tension. Relax, leaving your lips slightly parted.
8 Press your tongue against the roof of your mouth. Hold the tension. Relax, keeping your lips slightly parted.
9 Press your head back and notice the tension in your neck. Roll it to the right and hold the tension. Then roll it to the left and hold. Straighten your head and bring it forward, so it presses against your chest. Hold the tension. Relax.
10 Shrug your shoulders as if lifting them to your ears. Hold the tension. Relax. Breathe in deeply and hold it. Then let the air out. Repeat several times. Tighten your stomach but keep on breathing. Hold the tension. Relax.
11 Arch your back without straining. Feel the tension in the lower back. Hold the tension. Relax.
12 Tighten your buttocks and thighs by pressing down heels hard. Hold the tension. Relax.
13 Press your toes away from your face with your heels on the ground (if sitting), making your calves tense. Hold the tension. Relax.
14 Bend your toes up toward your face, with your heels on the ground, tensing your shins. Hold the tension. Relax.
15 Relax all over. Imagine a wave of relaxation starting from your toes, moving slowly through your entire body until it reaches the very top of the head. Enjoy the deep feeling of relaxation, warmth, and pleasure.

Making and using a 15 or 20 minute tape recording of the above technique may help. Many prerecorded tapes that make use of the progressive muscle relaxation technique exist.

Practise a preferred technique once or twice a day. Be sure to wait at least an hour after a meal before practising, otherwise the exercise may result in drowsiness. Remember to stay awake during the exercise. Its purpose is to achieve a relaxed state that both refreshes and ultimately energizes. If necessary, keep eyes open while practising. If unable to stay awake, practise with eyes open. It may be easier to sit and stay alert.

Meditation

Meditating is about finding and maintaining a quiet, peaceful attitude. When thoughts wander, it is fine to gently let them go and return to the breathing pattern and mantra (focus on a word or phrase). Begin meditating for about five to ten minutes, once or twice a day. After several weeks of regular meditation, do so for 15 or 20 minutes. To do this exercise, you will:

1 Find a quiet place where you can be alone and undisturbed.
2 Sit on a comfortable chair or on a pillow on the floor.
3 Close your eyes if that is what is most comfortable for you. If you are prone to falling asleep during meditation, stare at a place on the floor several feet in front of you. Keep that as your focal point.
4 Be quiet and peaceful, sitting quietly and following your breath. Don't force anything or deliberately try to slow your natural breathing pattern. Your breathing will slow naturally the further you go into the meditation.
5 As you exhale, allow your abdomen to gently rise and fall. As you do this, silently repeat a mantra such as "One," a name of God (Jesus, Allah, Jehovah, Buddha), "Relax", or any other word or phrase with a special meaning for you. You may repeat the word several times instead throughout the meditation for each time you inhale and exhale.

Visualization

Creating a pleasant image in the mind can calm and soothe jangled nerves and help relieve the stress of everyday cares. As you're doing this exercise, breathing becomes more relaxed and natural. Visualization is a particularly effective way to let go of negative thoughts. To do the exercise, you will:

1 Take the time to be alone and undisturbed.
2 Remove shoes and loosen any constricting clothing.
3 Lie down on a bed or couch, leaving hands and feet uncrossed.
4 Shut your eyes and focus them upward or downward, whatever feels best.
5 Breathe deeply for several minutes to let go of any excess tension. Let go of any thoughts distracting you. Focus on the present moment. Right now, in the moment, there is nothing you have to do and no place where you have to be. Do this for about two or three minutes in complete silence.
6 Begin the visualization. Imagine a place, perhaps a setting from the past where you were comfortable and happy or a place you have always wanted to visit. What does this setting look like? Are there other people around you or are you alone? What are some of the smells you're picking up? What sounds do you hear? Are you close to the water? Use all your senses and make the images as real as possible.
7 Notice that your breathing has become more relaxed and natural. As you continue to breathe, relaxingly, deeply, move yourself through your imaginary setting. View it from a number of angles. Continue to let go of any disturbing thoughts that arise. Feel the peacefulness that surrounds you.
8 Gradually re-alert yourself to your present surroundings. Count slowly from one to ten. Now slowly open your eyes.
9 Whenever you are ready, slowly sit up again.

Some audiotapes that the authors have used and recommend highly to our patients are:

- *Letting Go Of Stress* by Emmett Miller and Steven Halpern, 1–800–52–TAPES
- *Autogenics* by Intrinsic Development (self-hypnotic suggestions for relaxation), 1–800–354–2858
- *Wilderness Daydreams One, Canoe/Rain* (guided imagery), 1–800–247–6789

• *Time for Joy* by Ruth Fishel (pleasant imagery relaxation followed by affirmations), 1–800–441–5569

Practicing deep relaxation using one of the methods described above is not the same as relaxing while reading a favourite book or doing woodwork in the garage. Deep relaxation is a natural state in which blood pressure drops, muscles relax, breathing slows down and deepens, the heart slows down, and other recuperative changes take place.

Deep relaxation is the polar opposite of the stress response described by Hans Selye, an early leader in stress research. Daily practise of relaxation, meditation, or visualization develops feelings of general peace and calm by reducing anxiety, improving sleep, and reducing overall muscle tension. In addition, because stress is fatiguing, slowing down inwardly results in increased energy and feelings of well-being.

16

Keeping a Journal

For now we see through a mirror only, but then face to face. Now I know in part; then I shall understand fully, even as I have been fully understood.

1 Corinthians 13:12

In *Opening Up: The Healing Power of Confiding in Others*, James Pennebaker (1990) explains how writing about life experiences can improve physical and emotional health. He discovered that writing about traumatic experiences for as little as 15 minutes a day reduces visits to a physician, improves immune function, and enhances performance at work. He argues that holding back thoughts and feelings requires a lot of energy. Over time, this energy expenditure stresses the body. Putting emotions into words brings about catharsis and relief and can help a person find meaning within a complex situation. Pennebaker suggests that the person focusing on life experiences write:

- For about 20 minutes in a quiet place
- Non-stop, paying no attention to grammar, punctuation, spelling, or logic
- For himself or herself only, as it is much easier to be honest that way
- Planning to return to overwhelmingly painful subjects later
- Expecting the strong feelings and emotions that writing can elicit.

JS felt downhearted in the early part of 1998 and could not figure out why. Everything seemed to be going well: her office was running smoothly, she had a nice staff, a good group of patients, and a full private life. What was making her sad? Journaling helped her figure this out during a short vacation from work. She had an opportunity to go to San Francisco on business. She went alone a few days early, just to get in touch with her thoughts and feelings. Sometimes when she is with other people she finds it distracts her from self-examination. She walked the lovely paths in the Muir Redwoods and also along the coast of Sausalito as well as the two miles from her hotel to City Lights bookstore. She took a bike ride. And she wrote whatever came to mind in her journal. Without planning it, she wrote about aging. She was to turn 50 in a few months and this seemed to be what was making her sad.

She wrote about how turning 50 was harder for women than for men. She wrote that women are judged on their appearance as well as their intelligence. While in San Francisco she began to read books about turning 50 and came to realize that she was heading toward a time of great potential.

JS discovered that as long as she felt vital and growing, age did not matter. Journaling helped her identify the source of her sadness. When she did turn 50, instead of feeling regret she realized that a full life still stretched before her.

Ira Progoff commented in his helpful book *At a Journal Workshop* (1975) that persons attending workshops believed they experienced feelings of "profound prayer and deep meditation." He suggests that as they step back and move inward people can begin to solve life's problems by looking honestly at their conflicts, anxieties, grief, joys, and life decisions.

Progoff believes that "the purpose of exploration is neither to diagnose nor to judge but to enable our life to disclose to us what its goals and meanings are." As a person looks back at periods of happiness, despair, failures, and successes, she gradually begins to discover that life has been going somewhere, however unaware of it she may have been.

Progoff recommends keeping a log section and a feedback section in journals. The purpose of the log is to provide a source of material for use in other parts of the journal. The log section contains brief, factual entries about life's events, feelings, or dreams, which are presented neutrally, objectively, in everyday-language, in some detail but without elaboration. There is no need to write politely or elegantly, as a journal is not literature; it is not meant for the eyes of others. Above all, there need be no self-judgment and no censoring of memories associated with shame, because a healing aspect of self-expression is accepting whatever comes to mind. The best time to recount the day's events is at the end of each day, addressing some of the following questions:

- How did you feel physically in the day?
- Did you remember the dream you had the night before or at least part of it?
- What feelings, fantasies, and worries moved through your mind as you performed the tasks of the day?
- What kind of relationships did you experience today?
- Did you feel affection for someone?
- Were you angry? Envious? Jealous?

The feedback section of the journal asks the keeper of the journal to draw upon the content of daily life and then to go deeper, without intellectualizing or heavy analysis.

The Intern Blues: The Private Ordeals of Three Young Doctors by Robert Marion (1989) presents the private notes of three interns writing from July 1985 to June 1986. Here are two examples from journal entries that illustrate the feedback section:

Andy – Thursday, December 12, 1985
I don't think I've put much of an entry into this thing for a long time. I think I've made it out of my month or two of depression, and I haven't felt the need to vent about things as badly. Even though I still wind up cursing about life, and still hate being on call more than anything else I can ever remember hating, and I'm still chronically tired, I'm definitely not depressed anymore. I don't know why: maybe it's because I know vacation is coming up very soon. Maybe it's because I like working on 8 East because of the social feel of the place: It's as if the whole staff is part of one big family. I just don't know ...

I ran into Mike Miller the other day. When he said Hi to me, he kind of frowned. And I sort of frowned when I saw him frown. I said, "What's the face?" He said, "Well, I'm just sad you're going to be leaving and you're not going to be around here next year." I don't know if that's what he was frowning about. At any rate, it's a nice thing to say.

Amy – Sunday, June 15, 1986
Kara Smith died Friday night. She had developed a fever on Sunday. Ron was on, he examined her, and he thought she had pneumonia. He didn't do anything about it, just wrote a note documenting it in the chart. Then on

Friday during the day, her breathing became very laboured. She must have been hypoxic. I felt very uncomfortable. I kept coming into the room to check on her. I know she was D.N.R., but just sitting around doing nothing really bothered me. I wanted at least to get a blood gas and maybe start some oxygen, but the rules are no treatment ...

She finally stopped breathing about twelve-thirty. We covered her with her blanket and just walked out of the room.

I called her mother. I got her on the phone and told her that Kara had died. She seemed very composed. She asked if I thought Kara had felt any pain. I told her I didn't think so, that she had seemed comfortable the whole time. Then the mother said, "I guess she's up with the angels now," and that's when she started to cry. I couldn't think of anything to say ...

After we hung up, the rest of the evening was quiet; I didn't get any admissions, and the ward was calm. I went to the on-call room but I couldn't sleep. I kept thinking about Kara's mother.

(Marion, 1989)

Writing can lead to insights on how to live life. Hugh Prather's book *Notes to Myself* (1970) contains short passages that illuminate some aspects of living, such as:

- Many people think they are acting the way they feel when they tell someone off. Someone is critical of me and I answer by calling him an SOB. My feeling is not that he is an SOB; my feeling is that he has hurt me. "You have hurt my feelings and now I want to hurt yours." Launching a verbal attack covers up my feelings of being hurt with an appearance of strength. I get angry when I think someone has hurt me in a way I am helpless to do anything about.
- A sure way for me to have a disastrous experience is to do something because it will be good for me.

Journaling is an important way to develop a relationship with the self. The person writing a journal accepts feelings, explores experiences and values, and clarifies meanings. The authors recommend doctors write about their experiences without judgment on a regular basis, following Progoff's suggestions.

17

Spirituality

O divine Master
Grant that I may not so much seek
To be consoled as to console
To be understood as to understand
To be loved as to love:
For it is in giving that we receive;
It is in pardoning that we are pardoned;
It is in dying to self that we are born to eternal life.

The Prayer of St. Francis, Eknath Easwaran,
God Makes the Rivers to Flow:
Passages for Meditation, 1982

Many physicians find that spirituality enhances their emotional and physical health, whether or not they believe in a personal God or belong to an organized religion.

A sense of the spiritual can help a person better understand the meaning of life and care for others. There are many ways to break down the walls of the ego and become part of a bigger whole, spiritually speaking. Albert Einstein touched on this when he wrote:

A human being is part of the whole called by us 'universe,' a part limited in time and space. We experience ourselves, our thoughts and feelings, as something separate from the rest, a king of optical delusion of consciousness. This delusion is a kind of prison for us, restricting us to our personal desires and to affections for a few persons nearest to us. Our task must be to free ourselves from the prison by widening our circle of compassion to embrace all living creatures and the whole of nature in its beauty. (McFarlane, 2003: 35)

Spirituality defines how people discern meaning and purpose in their lives. Some people find deeper meaning in traditional ways by participating in organized religion while others enter a path of self-discovery and experimentation apart from organized religion. (In chapter 9, "The Spiritual Needs of Children Who Are Dying," the authors discuss the concept of spirituality and how it contrasts with religion in more detail.)

Organized religions, including Protestantism, Judaism, Islam, and Buddhism, offer moral laws, dogmas, traditions, and behavioral expectations; they also assume obedience from their participants. The best way for many is the religion of childhood, if it offers memories, comfort, shared values, inspiration, and a sense of purpose. A physician whom AC treated wanted help with his anger outbursts. He exploded frequently at his staff, patients, and his own family. He was very traditional, valued authority, and was inspired by and respected the teachings of his church. Though he was not actively involved when he first came to AC, he decided to strengthen his church ties. This reconnection helped him to find the way to manage his frequent outbursts and judgmental attitude toward others.

Other people see themselves as seekers, who search through the spiritual traditions of the world, hoping to find a path that resonates with their own experience and values. Bookstores, conferences, audiotapes, retreats, and places of worship provide access to many traditions, beliefs, and practices, which can be exhilarating or very confusing to the seeker.

Within the traditional religions there are mystical paths as well, for example, Sufism within Islam, Kabala within Judaism, and Tibetan Buddhism within Buddhism. As John Lash points out in *The Seeker's Handbook* (1990), seekers today may be guided by a desire for self-discovery and self-guidance but may end up identifying with alternative beliefs and rituals that can be as strict as the ones in the religion of their upbringing.

However, some people prefer to maintain their independence and identify with a religious tradition without accepting all its precepts or participating in all its rituals. AC, for example, was born into a Jewish family but attended Catholic school while a child in Cuba. In spite of Jewish instruction and synagogue attendance as a teenager, he found himself drawn to books about Buddhism. Over the years his interest in Buddhist principles and spiritual practises deepened, although he had little interest in becoming a member of any temple or meditation centre. These beliefs now guide him in his encounters with human suffering. He sees his beliefs as a system for living, not as a religion.

SOME WAYS TO NURTURE SPIRITUALITY

There are many ways to experience the sacred. Some people already belong to a church or temple, which brings a feeling of community and support to spiritual longings. Twelve-step support groups, Bible study groups, and regular meetings with others to share thoughts, feelings, and dreams can also provide the social context to nourish spiritual needs.

Reading the Bible, the Koran, other sacred literature, or inspirational books on a regular basis, listening to inspirational music, watching movies with spiritual themes, or looking at great art can also help people access the spiritual within themselves.

Many people find that regular prayer, meditation practises, and spending time alone or with one other person in the woods, mountains, or by an ocean or lake to be revitalizing experiences. Such experiences remind them of the truth Albert Einstein put so well in the passage quoted earlier. Everything is interconnected. The ordinary world is sacred.

Gain Inspiration through Books

The authors recommend reading something that inspires or touches the soul for at least half an hour every night before going to sleep. The lives of others unfold in a book, so that a reader can share their thoughts, feelings, and dreams. As the characters solve their problems, the reader can learn from their experience, see life more clearly, make decisions, and gain courage. The book may even inspire readers to change. Some books offer uplifting ideas and practical suggestions for living well.

Following are the titles (with other details in the References section) of some books the authors recommend to help readers access their spiritual side:

The Big Book of Alcoholics Anonymous, fourth edition. This book, which was written in 1939 when AA had only 100 members, discusses the twelve steps of AA, providing clear, concise steps on how to implement the steps into daily life. A physician who was one of the founders of AA wrote sizable portions of this book.

It contains many inspirational stories as well – stories that are heartfelt and still ring true today. AA offers a very healing program for many people. Physicians who don't have a problem with alcohol abuse may want to read this book to get a clearer picture of what alcoholism is all about.

Being Peace by Thich Nhat Hanh, a Buddhist monk, who writes about living peacefully in the present moment. While in Vietnam during the war, he saw many people die painful deaths. Through that experience he developed an enormous amount of compassion, compassion that is reflected in all his writing.

My Own Country by Abraham Verghese, a doctor, who writes about treating patients who were HIV positive during the early part of the AIDS epidemic. With admirable honesty, Verghese describes how his being with these people affected his own life and the lives of his family members.

Death Be Not Proud by John Gunther. The author describes how his son learned he had brain cancer and how the family and his son handled the treatments. Many of the treatments were alternative; at the time Gunther wrote the book, modern medicine had little to offer these patients except surgery. Gunther also describes the moment his son died. Gunther's honesty encouraged JS to become a physician.

How We Die: Reflections on Life's Final Chapter by Sherwin B. Nuland, a surgeon who frankly, yet compassionately, tells how most people are likely to die. He describes the dying mechanism of cancer, heart attacks, strokes, AIDS, and Alzheimer's disease. Any physician, nurse, or health care professional will find this book worth reading.

My Own Story by Ryan White, who learned he had AIDS when he was just 13. Ryan described how this illness affected him and his family. He was forbidden to go to school with other children and had to go to court to win his right to attend. Ryan had a profound and rare wisdom. This wonderful book is easy to enjoy.

The Story of Josh by Marcia Friedman. Josh Friedman was only 20 when he was diagnosed with malignant brain cancer, a type of cancer that at the time was incurable. Josh showed great courage and strength. His doctor advised him to have surgery immediately but because Josh wisely thought that brain surgery might impair his thinking, he took some time before he had the surgery to take care of matters that were important to him. Finally, when the pain became unbearable, he asked to end his life with a morphine drip. His doctor, although he denied he was involved in assisted suicide, helped him. The authors do not agree with assisted suicide, but this book makes a good case for it. Josh, though just a young adult, was in control of his life and his medical treatment.

Here are some other books worth reading:

The Bible
The Dhammapada
It's Not About the Bike: My Journey Back to Life by Lance Armstrong
The Denial of Death by Ernest Becker
The Wisdom of No Escape by Pema Chodron
Meditation: A Simple Eight-Point Program for Translating Spiritual Ideas into Daily Life by Eknath Easwaran
Take Your Time by Eknath Easwaran
Chop Wood, Carry Water, edited by Rick Fields.
The Prophet by Kahlil Gibran
The Miracle of Mindfulness by Thich Nhat Hanh
On Death and Dying by Elisabeth Kübler-Ross
When Bad Things Happen to Good People by Rabbi Harold Kushner
Notes to Myself: My Struggle to Become a Person by Hugh Prather
It's Always Something by Gilda Radner
Kitchen Table Wisdom: Stories that Heal by Rachel Naomi Remen
AIDS and Its Metaphors by Susan Sontag
Illness as a Metaphor by Susan Sontag
Gratefulness, the Heart of Prayer by David Steindl-Rast
Shambhala: The Sacred Path of the Warrior by Chogyam Trungpa
Saint Maybe by Anne Tyler

Gain Inspiration through Films

Films serve a multitude of purposes. A comedy can bring a person laughter and respite from the day's problems. Films about culture, personal events, and tragedies can help a person understand another point of view or have empathy for another's situation. They can also help a person understand a different time and place. Some inspirational films follow.

Harold and Maude. Harold (Bud Cort), a young man who is bored with his wealth but very interested in death, likes to go to funerals. While at a funeral, he meets Maude (Ruth Gordon), who sees only people's good intentions and really loves life. She teaches Harold, who becomes her much younger lover, how to enjoy living again.

Fearless. An architect (Jeff Bridges) survives an airplane crash and is transformed. He loses his fear of danger of all kinds and becomes strangely alienated from the rest of humanity. This serious movie is about the nature of fear and its relationship to being human.

Wit. A scholarly English professor (Vivian Bearing), whose field is the poetry of John Donne, is diagnosed with Stage 4 ovarian cancer. While she undergoes full-strength highly toxic chemotherapy, the doctors and residents treat her as if she were merely an interesting object of research. Without compassion or kindness, they subject her to tests and exams of various sorts. She realizes she did not think kindness mattered when she was dealing with her students. The story also touches on DNR orders and pain control issues. The physicians are two-dimensional, but the performances and writing are of high caliber and the film is riveting.

Gain Inspiration through Music

Music can calm emotions, focus attention, and even help release negative thoughts. Because of its power, music can become a favourite source of encouragement and support. Some readers might enjoy:

Alleluia: On the Wings of Song. The chanting by Robert Gass, using Bach's music is hypnotic and soothing, as are other chants by Gass.

Annie. The heartening musical is, of course, based on the long running comic strip about an orphan girl who finds a home, love, and security.

A Chorus Line. This musical, in which people tell their stories about struggling to become dancers on Broadway, is very uplifting.

Passages. A modern experimental composer, Philip Glass, and a classical Indian musician, Ravi Shankar, joined forces to create a melodic and spiritual symphony.

Here is some other inspirational music:

Ave Maria: Meditation, Joel Andrews
The Eternal Om, Robert Slap (producer)
A Feather on the Breath of God, Hildegard de Bingen.
Gloria: On Wings of Song, Robert Gass
Narada World: A Global Vision (Vol. 1 and 2), various artists
Pachelbel Canon, Bach
Pure Moods, various artists
Shepherd Moons and Watermark, Enya
Songs of Sanctuary, Adiemus
Yeha-Noha, Sacred Spirits

SOURCES OF SUPPORT

Physicians who have had the chance to review a number of ideas and suggestions in this chapter may now take a few minutes to list a few of the suggestions they might want to try. Some might pick up a book or piece of music suggested above, enjoying their choice during a quiet evening at home. Others may be motivated to begin a journal or take up a sport in which they have long been interested.

Perhaps some just need to call a friend or write a letter to someone they haven't heard from in a long time. Whatever they choose, they need to choose something replenishing, something that enhances their well-being. If they think they don't have time to relax, *Take Your Time* by Eknath Easwaran (1994) will provide some ideas.

Physicians expend a lot of energy taking care of others and making sure their needs are met on a daily basis. Unfortunately, they often forget that they need the same kind of care and attention. They, too, have the right to seek emotional and inspirational support and to make sure that when they fall ill, they are cared for with compassion and gentleness during their illness and during the often gloomy time that follows.

18

Opening Up to Others

A friend is a person with whom I may be sincere. Before him I may think aloud.

Ralph Waldo Emerson (1803–1882)

A dying patient, especially one who is young, can cause emotional turmoil for a physician. JS took care of a man in his early twenties who died, in part, because he had not taken his antiviral medications on a regular basis. At times he would take the medications faithfully, then he would become discouraged and stop. Eventually he became resistant to all antivirals; he had a rising viral load and a very low CD4 count. His resistance to life-threatening illness was almost non-existent. JS felt a great deal of guilt about this patient's illness and his failure to take his medications. She felt much sadness, but did not know why.

Sharing thoughts, feelings, emotions, and struggles within an atmosphere of mutual support offers many healthy rewards. Those who open up to others will:

GET TO KNOW THEMSELVES BETTER

People know themselves to the extent that they make themselves known. Often their thoughts, feelings, and needs remain vague and cloudy until they put them into words. Asking others to understand what they feel, think, and want can make things much clearer for them. Of course, thoughts and feelings may sometimes conflict. When people talk about themselves they bring this conflict into the open.

A surgeon who had put in the central line for a young patient of JS told her that he felt very sad every time he saw the young man. When she asked why, he explained that the patient's medical record troubled him, because here was a young man who might have survived if he had just taken his medication. Another doctor felt sad about the young man's shame over being HIV positive and regretted that his religion did not allow him to accept that part of himself. He felt that the young man's religious views, not lack of information, had been the cause of his non-compliance.

Talking to these two physicians helped JS realize that her rational thoughts were in conflict with her feelings. Rationally, she realized she didn't have the power to make the young man comply. What she felt was not so much guilt as sadness for a life gone far too soon.

GET TO KNOW OTHER PEOPLE BETTER

When people tell others about their feelings and thoughts, the others grow more comfortable doing the same. When that happens, trust grows. When trust grows, friendships can deepen.

FEEL LESS GUILT

Guilt is a feeling with two parts. People may feel anger because they did something or failed to do something – or just thought something. They may then fear punishment, which is always painful to feel and often undeserved.

Talking about oneself can often relieve guilt. When anger and fear are out in the open, people can look at themselves with more clarity. They can get honest feedback from other people and judge whether the guilt is neurotic or offers an opportunity to apologize and make amends.

Guilt may occur when people follow restrictive rules and beliefs so closely that they often say:

- If I ask for help, I'll look weak.
- If I try hard enough, then I can succeed at everything.
- If I can't do this perfectly, then I won't do it at all.

Talking about these feelings helps people discover and "unlearn" such restrictive beliefs. They gain energy because hiding thoughts and feelings absorbs energy. Feelings that stay stuffed inside a person tend to simmer and then explode in unpredictable ways. Talking about these emotions relieves the pressure decreasing the likelihood of lashing out and possibly hurting oneself and others.

LEARN TO TALK ABOUT THEMSELVES

This may sound like the easiest thing in the world to do. "I do it all the time," we might say. Actually, some ways of sharing thoughts and feelings support happiness and spiritual growth more than others do. Some of the following suggestions may be helpful. When doing this a person may:

- Choose a good place to talk, a quiet, comfortable and inviting place where there will be few interruptions. Some settings promote good communication while others prevent it. Trying to talk with someone in a noisy office, where the phone rings every few minutes, is usually frustrating.
- Share something new. Talk about something that's fresh – possibly something that's happened that very day. To become more skillful at talking about oneself requires talking about new subjects rather than tired information everyone's already heard before.
- Be honest. Talking about oneself requires honesty. If you are being less than honest, people are usually savvy enough to pick up on this and tune out very quickly.
- Notice the response of the listener. Watch his face, eyes, and body movement. Is he asking questions and giving feedback? Does he look concerned and interested? If not, consider ending the conversation or switching the topic.
- Talk about death and dying. Sharing these feelings can be tricky for physicians. To avoid getting hurt, they might begin by giving only the facts – who was involved, what happened, and where and how it happened. If comfortable, they may then go beyond and beneath the facts to talk about the impact of the death of a particular patient on them. They may share their desire to be comfortable about the topic. Finally, they may consider asking others for help, as many just need a request to be supportive. Doctors may ask if they can call others when they find themselves feeling low or when they just want to talk.
- Stay in the here and now. Talking about oneself takes practise. It always helps to stay in the "now." Those who talk about how they feel at the moment and who admit a subject makes them uneasy or that they feel scared, embarrassed, or fearful will make their listeners feel trusted and help draw them closer.

Doctors can open themselves to people other than colleagues, perhaps to their spouses or best friends. Talking is therapeutic, keeps relationships alive and growing, and promotes self-understanding. Doctors will find it very helpful to choose one person with whom they can share their problems and joys of the day, someone who is

- Not judgmental
- A good listener
- Accepting, allowing them to progress at their own pace
- Not a "fixer-upper," that is, a person who makes frequent suggestions and becomes angry when others disagree or choose not to follow their advice.
- Understanding about the emotions involved or willing to ask for clarification when confused.

The authors suggest the following exercise:

- Talk about your day's events to your spouse or best friend or the person described above each day for about 10 to 15 minutes
- Listen to them for an equal amount of time as they talk about their day.

Some doctors may find themselves at a loss as to what to talk about. It's productive, though, to talk about:

- The best moment of the day
- Something upsetting that happened that day
- Something funny or sad that happened that day
- A spiritual or personal insight.

People will find it much easier to talk than they thought if they:

- Express compliments and appreciation openly.
- Spend a few moments writing down a few things people did for them during the day that they appreciated.
- Think about what other physicians, nurses, and support staff did to help during the day and then tell them that. While JS was an intern, she was supervised by a resident who never spoke to

her about her work – never even said hello. He was shocked one evening when JS went off to sit by herself during dinner at the cafeteria, because he was amazed that she didn't even consider him a friend. It turns out that he had many good thoughts about her; he just never expressed them.

- Get thoughts out of their heads, simply by expressing them.
- Not fear their own emotional responses, even of crying. They'll understand themselves better.

Physicians live in a difficult and stressful world. Besides dealing with death and dying, they must often accept unfair rules and regulations. They need all the compassion they can get and will help their colleagues if they express their compassion to them.

19

Leading a Balanced Life

Be aware of wonder. Live a balance life – learn some and think some and draw and paint and sing and dance and play and work every day some.

Robert Fulghum, *All I Really Need to Know I Learned in Kindergarten*, 1989.

When the authors were in college, they were often asked if they felt "centered." They never really knew what the word meant until they read *Centering in Pottery, Poetry, and the Person* by Mary Caroline Richards (1989). She wrote that when the clay is centered on the rotating potter's wheel, the potter will make a perfect pot. If too much clay is on one side or the other, the pot will fall. Human lives are like that clay on the wheel. If there is too much of any one thing, life will be out of balance; it will fall.

A healthy lifestyle includes and balances work, play, exercise, spiritual growth, family, friends, and rest. This balanced lifestyle is often very difficult for a physician to achieve, given the demands of the profession, especially in residency. For example, the authors know a man whose wife went through an especially hectic residency; she and her husband rarely saw one another. Even today, with a thriving practise and staff, they're often ships passing in the night. The man jokes on occasion "We've made an appointment to have sex on April 23, 2010 at 3:00 PM. If her four o'clock cancels, we may get more than an hour." While humorous, the situation must also be quite painful at times.

Time management can help physicians maintain a balance. In the book *The Seven Habits of Highly Effective People*, Stephen Covey (1989) suggest his readers arrange their time based on their values.

Each reader completes what is most important first and then eliminates the tasks that fall outside those values.

Doctors can decrease stress by determining what they have time for and what they really want to do. A physician friend of the authors, who was having medical problems, felt very stressed. When her close friends or relatives had a medical problem, they asked her to participate in their care. She told us that she simplified her life by asking herself why she was doing what she was doing. If she wanted to do something, she would consider taking it on or continuing the obligation. If she did not want to do it, she didn't. She also asked herself if she could afford to do the project physically and emotionally, and if she had the time to do it. If she could not answer yes, she declined. She suddenly found her life simpler and less stressful. She was also amazed at how much her health improved.

The daily choices that physicians must make and the activities in which they are involved can obscure their goals. When JS was a resident she met an internist who had graduated from college and medical school at an early age. He told her he believed he would die young because his father had. He decided to live his life at a rapid speed so that he would not miss anything. He got married, had children, and owned his own home before he had finished his residency. He even moonlighted to pay off his medical school loans. One day he collapsed from emotional exhaustion. He admitted to a friend that he had taken on too much and just could not do it all anymore. He then decided to determine what was most important to him. In his case, it was his wife and children. He restructured his life to be with them more. He is alive and well and has outlived his father.

An unbalanced life can be a sign of an underlying problem. A physician whom JS knew as an intern put in 12 to 15 hour days at the hospital. JS thought he was simply hardworking but he was actually having marriage problems. Working long hours allowed him to avoid his problems at home. When he resolved his marriage problems, he didn't have to work as many hours.

Another physician whom the authors know experienced the death of a family member. He never cried or grieved and did not spend time with his wife and children. He just seemed to work to avoid his grief. He believed that if he started crying he would never stop. Being an anesthesiologist, he worked on as many cases as he could and made a great deal of money. Actually he was also working long hours to have access to drugs that he used in his work. Eventually he did get help. He went to many NA meetings and gave many lectures on sobriety. Unfortunately, although he is still sober, he continues to put his family second.

If doctors find themselves spending too much time working or in some other activity, they may ask themselves about the underlying reason. Are they trying to avoid a personal problem or feeling? Do they have a drug or alcohol problem they are trying to hide?

When health care providers work long hours, they simply do not have time to develop their spiritual side. Spirituality is often developed when they can be alone with their thoughts. As Eknath Easwaran states in *Take Your Time: Finding Balance in a Hurried World* (1994), when people slow down their pace of life, they allow themselves to live in the present and to enjoy important things.

Doctors, then, may ask themselves when they last really listened to their children or other loved ones, noticed the clouds in the sky or the smell in the air after the rain. When people are faced with their own mortality, they often wish they had taken the time to enjoy life's simple pleasures. Enjoying the spirituality of simplicity comes from being centered and having balance. As Thich Nhat Hanh writes in *Peace Is Every Step*: "Peace is present right here and now, in ourselves and in everything we do and see. The question is whether or not we are in touch with it" (Nhat Hanh, 1991: 5). Enjoying what happens from moment to moment can be the foundation for a healthy spiritual life.

Taking time allows for prayer and meditation. Those who take time to be quiet and still can also listen to their own thoughts and feelings and come to know themselves better. By listening to their thoughts and feelings, they can learn to live with themselves and even how to love themselves.

Taking time can also allow people to attend to their own physical well-being. Doctors tell patients to watch their cholesterol, to diet, and to exercise. How many physicians tend to their own advice? JS was never athletic in school. In fact, when teams were chosen she was generally the last one picked. Several years ago, though, she took up bike riding and speed walking and began to feel fit for the first time in her life. She also has an exercise program that she follows and she plans the week ahead with plenty of fruits, vegetables, rice, and grains on hand. In her diet and exercise log books, she writes down long-term and short-term goals and records her progress. This is her way of managing her time, exercise, and diet. Looking at these records helps her identify stress points in her life.

Why exercise and have a sound diet? First, it promotes health. For instance, a woman who exercises and maintains her weight has a lower risk of breast cancer. Both men and women find that exercise decreases their risk of heart disease and diabetes.

More important, exercising and caring for one's body can also be a spiritual practice. Being aware of and maintaining the body (as well as the mind) is a spiritual act of self-love. Everyone has the right to love and care for themselves.

Family is an important part of developing a balanced life. It is especially important for people who work in the health care professions, where the hours are long and down time is often very little. How do they keep from shutting out their families during that minimal down time?

The brother-in-law of a former editor of the authors runs a very successful dental practise in Florida, where he has been based for over 20 years and where he employs nearly ten people. For many years this dentist spent countless hours at work, as he built his practise. Yet, his wife and two children were very important to him. He knew that his children's early years were important ones developmentally and he wanted to be with them as much as possible. He decided to end his workweek at noon on Friday, leaving him two and a half days to spend with his family each week. His gesture and his commitment to it revealed his love to his children. Our former editor still admires his brother-in-law for doing that, because it reveals much about him and his priorities.

A balanced life includes a healthy mix of work, exercise, eating, family and friends, leisure activities, spiritual practise, and sleep. To be healthy, health care providers need to find a balance among these parts of life.

THE BALANCE WHEEL

To help you see if you are spending your time as you would like, fill in the 24-hour wheel. How many hours each day do you spend:

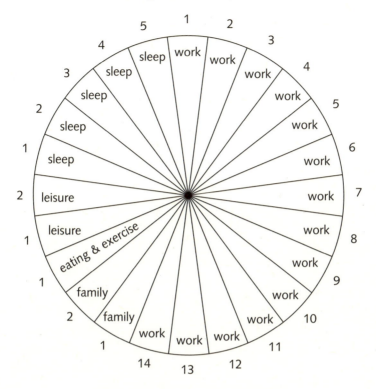

Figure 1: Joe's Actual 24-hour Wheel

- Working?
- Sleeping?
- Eating?
- Exercising?
- On spiritual health?
- On leisure activities?
- With your family?

For example, Joe, a cardiologist answered these questions this way:

- Working?   14
- Sleeping?   5
- Eating?   0.5
- Exercising?   0.5

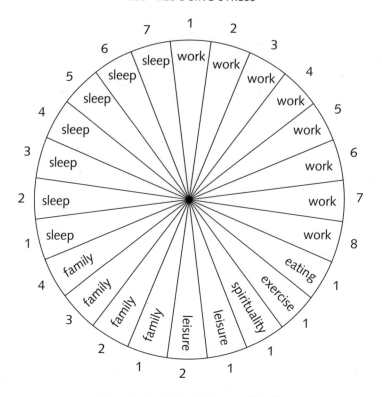

Figure 2: Joe's Ideal 24-hour Wheel

- On spiritual health?   o
- On leisure activities?   2
- With your family?   2

When asked if he was satisfied with the wheel, he answered no. He then redid the wheel as he would like it to be.

- Working?   8
- Sleeping?   7
- Eating?   1
- Exercising?   1
- On spiritual health?   1
- On leisure activities?   2
- With your family?   4

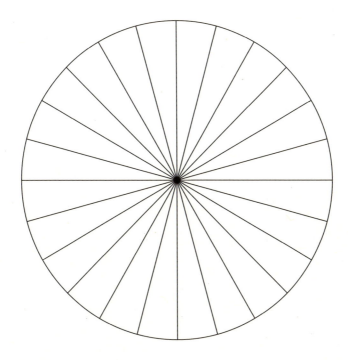

Figure 3: Your Actual 24-hour Wheel

Now fill in the 24-hour wheel for yourself. How many hours each day do you spend:

- Working?
- Sleeping?
- Eating?
- Exercising?
- On spiritual health?
- On leisure activities?
- With your family?

Are you satisfied with this wheel? Please redo the wheel as you would like it to be. How many hours each day do you ideally spend?

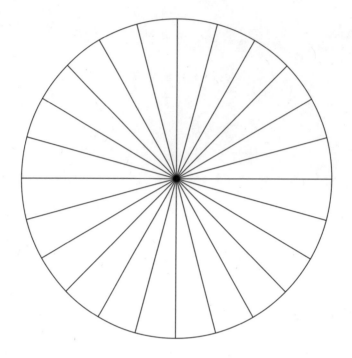

Figure 4: Your Ideal 24-hour Wheel

- Working?
- Sleeping?
- Eating?
- Exercising?
- On spiritual health?
- On leisure activities?
- With your family?

How could you achieve this new allocation of time?

1

2

3

4

EXERCISE

One effective way to reduce stress and fight depression is through exercise. Sports medicine expert, Kenneth Cooper, recommends the following guidelines (www.cooperaerobics.com):

- Achieve an age-appropriate balance between aerobic exercise and strength training. As a general guideline, Cooper recommends 20 to 30 minutes of aerobic activity, at least three to five times a week, and a 20-minute weight training session, which can include hand-held weights, machines, or calisthenics, at least twice a week.
- Choose an exercise program that will interest you. This can be brisk walking, jogging, cycling, bowling, or swimming. For weight training, choose a reputable fitness centre or hire a personal trainer.

OTHER WAYS TO RECHARGE

When physicians work in health care, they are continually putting the lives of others before their own. They decide their patients' medical paths and plan for their treatment, while the patients often put a tremendous amount of trust in their medical expertise and judgment. As caregivers, they must learn to care for themselves by taking the time daily to rejuvenate themselves.

Recharging is a time when they can focus on their needs and block out the needs of others, if only for a while. This personal time can reinvigorate their energy levels and general feeling of well being so that they can care for others as well. Ideally, they should put away the beeper and cell phone and ask not to be called. While on vacation, they should let covering doctors care for their patients and try not to check in. This is their own time. To recharge a person may enjoy a:

- Daily stretching routine
- Hot baths, saunas, and hot tubs
- Massages, by a professional or spouse
- A positive addiction. William Glasser (1976) wrote that a regular activity can become addictive in that you look forward to it and

miss it if you are not able to do it. Unlike negative addictions, these bring a person greater feelings of relaxation, physical well being, self-confidence, and a greater ability to cope with stress. Positive addictions have the following characteristics. They can be done:
- Easily with little mental effort
- Alone or with others, but do not depend on others
- Without criticizing oneself
- With gradual, subjective improvement

And they:
- Are non-competitive
- Require as little as an hour a day
- Are valuable to the person in physical, mental, or spiritual ways.
- TV, magazines, or other activity for an hour a day
- Time spent on the weekend, alone or with someone else, on a fun activity such as:

• Shopping	• Writing Poems
• Hiking	• Bird watching
• Bicycling	• Doing Yoga
• Reading	• Bowling
• Fishing	• Restoring antiques
• Doing carpentry	• Writing letters
• Playing golf	• Going to pet shows
• Taking photos	• Growing house plants
• Buying art objects	• Going to movies

Or whatever you used to enjoy or always meant to do when you had the time. Do it now.
- An extended weekend (three to four days) trip to a nearby destination.
- At least one entire week off every six months, spent in a place where it is easy to unwind and get away from daily stresses.

Thich Nhat Hanh wrote in *Peace Is Every Step*: "Every morning when we wake up, we have twenty-four brand new hours to live. What a precious gift! We have the capacity to live in a way that these twenty-four hours will bring peace, joy and happiness to ourselves and others" (Nhat Hanh, 1991: 5).

When doctors work with dying patients, they understand how precious an extra 24 hours can be to them and their families. Actually, every 24 hours can be important to everyone. By living a balanced life, every 24 hours can be precious and meaningful. Each and everyone can live each moment to its fullest, mindfully aware of themselves, their world, its people, and their loved ones.

Evaluating each day to see whether it is made up of a healthy mix of work, exercise, eating time, family time, leisure activities, spiritual practise, and sleep is an important exercise. The authors suggest allotting time to these activities in amounts that will bring increased energy and satisfaction.

Epilogue

The doctor is the familiar of death. When patients call for a doctor, they are asking him to cure them, but, if he cannot cure, the patients are also asking the doctor to witness them dying. The value of the witness is that he has seen so many others die. He is the living intermediary between us and the multitudinous dead. He belongs to us and he has belonged to them. And the hard but real comfort which they offer through him is that of fraternity.

John Berger, *A Fortunate Man: The Story of a Country Doctor,* 1981

Being a doctor is a gift. Doctors are there when a person is born and when he or she dies. They share in the patient's most intimate moments and know the patient's fears and hopes. This is the gift from their patients. By learning how to handle these difficult times and by learning to listen and talk to their patients, doctors can learn about others and themselves and take full advantage of this gift.

The authors of *A Physician's Guide to Coping with Death and Dying* have attempted to lay a foundation upon which physicians can build a caring and compassionate way to deal with their patients who are dying and their families. Part One examines death and dying and the six stages of dying that a physician will witness. The authors have identified six stages of dying: *Recognition, The Process of Dying, The Moment of Death, The Departure of the Spirit or Life Force, Terminal Care of the Body,* and *Dealing With Grief and Loss.* Health care providers can learn about these stages and help the patient and their families and loved ones deal with each stage effectively.

Part Two considers communication issues. How does a doctor talk to a patient who is dying? How does he discuss where and with whom the patient wants to die? How does a doctor discuss living wills and medical powers of attorney? How does she broach the topic of treatment or no treatment? How can doctors help patients and themselves face fears of death?

Part Three focuses on difficult situations, including death and dying in the ED, the problems of children who are dying or who have had a relative or close friend die, and the unique problems of physician-patients.

The last part of the book addresses how physicians can take care of themselves. How can they handle death in a positive manner while dealing with the issues of grief, sadness, and guilt that the death of a patient may arouse? The authors discuss how physicians can identify in themselves some illnesses and problems, including insomnia, alcohol abuse, and depression and address these in a constructive way. They discuss, too, how doctors can open themselves up to others and lead a balanced life so that they may better care for themselves while caring for their patients.

The readers of this book, who are experts in medical treatment, can also become experts in dealing with dying and death. By facing fears and biases, doctors can become self-aware and this awareness can give their patients strength and comfort. The authors know, too, how difficult it can be to follow through some of what they have suggested in this book. They realize that there will be times when doing so will not be humanly possible.

This book may be a stepping-stone for further reading and research about death and dying, as well as a tool for personal growth. The authors wish doctors and other health care professionals good luck in their valuable work with dying patients and their families!

To end on as upbeat a note as possible, the authors acknowledge that death is an end. At the same time, they suggest that the dying, their families, and their physicians can still grow as death approaches. Dying can put in focus what is important and bring people closer to others.

Resources

General Sources
  Medical Information
  On Death and Dying
Specific Sources
  Caregivers
  Children and Death and Dying
  Diseases and Disorders
    AIDS
    Arthritis
    Cancer
    Dementia
    Diabetes
    Digestive Diseases
    Heart Disease
    Kidney Diseases
    Neurological Diseases
    Pulmonary Diseases
    Sleep Disorders
  Medical Organizations
  Mental Heath Organizations
  Other Professional Organizations
    Ethics
    Pain, Palliative Care, Critical Care

There are numerous organizations available to physicians and their patients. In the local phone book, look under headings such as child treatment centres, cancer treatment centres, senior citizens services and organizations, social service organizations, AIDS information and services, crisis intervention services or under disease names such as "diabetes." These organizations may be able to provide information about related organizations in your area. The World Wide Web is also a wonderful resource. The authors have looked at a wide variety of websites in order to make some recommendations that they hope will be useful.

In the list of resources that follows, the section on death and dying lists organizations that provide a wide range of services from living wills to professional education for physicians to inexpensive funerals. The list of disease-specific organizations includes organizations that provide emotional support to individuals afflicted with the disease, disease specific information, and information on clinical trials. Some even offer financial help to patients. The section on children lists organizations dealing with the special needs of this population. Sections on professional organizations, grief resources, and help for caregivers are also included.

Websites listed here are often linked to other websites that provide additional and related information.

GENERAL SOURCES

Some interesting and useful general medical databases and reference sites include:
www.medlineplus.gov
www.locatorplus.gov
www.medscape.com
content.nejm.org
www.ncbi.nlm.nih.gov/gquery/gquery.fcgi
www.ncbi.nlm.nih.gov/entrez/query.fcgi

Medical Information

Med Help
www.medhelp.org
6300 North Wickham Rd., Suite 130, PMB #188, Melbourne, FL 32940
Phone: 321-259-7505
This non-profit organization website, which was founded to assist those in need of medical information, is written in non-technical language.

Healthfinder
www.healthfinder.gov
P.O. Box 1133, Washington, DC 20013-1133
Healthfinder provides consumer healthcare information from the US government, with selected online publications, databases, websites, and support groups.

On Death and Dying

Americans for Better Care of the Dying
www.abcd-caring.org
3720 Upton St. NW, Room B147, Washington, DC 20016
Phone: 202-895-2660
ABCD is a public non-profit organization dedicated to social, professional, and policy reform aimed at improving the care system for patients with serious illness and their families. It offers a voice to the many organizations, associations, and individuals committed to the idea that each person should have the opportunity to live meaningfully to the end.

Some of its recent web articles are "Handbook for Mortals: Guidance for People Facing Serious Illness," "MediCaring," "Agitator's Guide: Twelve Steps to Get Your Community Talking about Dying," "20 Improvements in End-of-Life Care – Changes Internists Could Do Next Week!" and "Potential Medicare Reimbursements for Services to Patients with Chronic Fatal Illnesses".

Bereaved Families Online Support Centre
www.bereavedfamilies.net
Bereaved Families of Ontario
36 Eglington Avenue West, Suite 602, Toronto, ON M4R 1A1
Phone: 416-440-0290
The mission of Bereaved Families of Ontario is to help the bereaved live with grief and find healing. This site has a column entitled Good Grief, an online library, reviews of books dealing with grief and healing, and links to related sites.

They provide group programs for children (age three and up) and adults and also offer custom programs for communities and workplaces affected by grief. Seminars, conferences, educational workshops, and a speaker's bureau are also available.

Bereavement Services and Support
www.bereavement.net
18 Suter Crescent. Dundas, ON L9H 6R5
Phone: 905-628-6008
Bereavement Services provides professional grief counselling and support services in the Golden Horseshoe Area of Ontario, Canada. The organization offers support groups (free of charge), educational seminars, and workshops for the bereaved and those wanting to learn more about the grieving process. The website has an order form for colouring books for grieving children for use in helping them cope better.

Canadian Hospice Palliative Care Association
www.chpca.net
43 Bruyere Street, Suite 131C, Ottawa, ON K1N 5C8
Phone: 613-241-3663 or 1-800-688-2785
GlaxoWellcome Info Line: 1-877-203-4636
A national organization that provides leadership to palliative care providers. It hopes to increase awareness, knowledge, and skills related to quality palliative care. The organization is developing national standards for hospice palliative care in Canada and supports research in palliative care.

The Canadian Virtual Hospice
www.canadianvirtualhospice.ca
One Morley Avenue, Room PE450, Administration Building
Winnipeg, MB R3H 2P4
Phone: 204-475-1494 or 1-866-288-4803
This internet-based network hopes to provide mutual support for Canadians affected by end-of-life issues. The site hopes to encourage the exchange of information and communication among healthcare professionals, palliative care researchers, and the terminally ill and their families.

Death in America, Project on Death, Dying, and Bereavement
www.soros.org/death.html
Project on Death in America, Open Society Institute
400 West 59th Street, New York, NY 10019
Phone: 212-548-0150
This site connects to a broad network of organizations involved in public education and policy, with an emphasis on expanding the dialogue

surrounding death and bereavement. In addition to its support for public and professional education efforts through its Grants Program, PDIA serves as a resource centre for the media, providing reporters and editors with information and assistance, including access to the PDIA network of experts on issues surrounding dying and grieving. The on-line PDIA Library Catalog contains approximately 600 documents on books, non-governmental organization reports, and videos concerned with such topics as death and dying, bereavement, grief, mourning, and palliative care.

The communication activities of PDIA help expand knowledge and coverage of dying issues beyond the debate of physician-assisted suicide. It is also very concerned with death in prisons.

Funeral Consumers Alliance
www.funerals.org
33 Patchen Road, South Burlington, VT 05403
Phone: 1-800-765-0107
The Funeral Consumers Alliance is dedicated to a consumer's right to choose a meaningful, dignified, affordable funeral. The site has a directory of nonprofit funeral consumer groups and also provides information on caring for the body after death and on body and organ donation.

The Growth House
www.growthhouse.org
Phone 415-863-3045
The Growth House is a comprehensive international gateway to resources on the web that are related to life-threatening illnesses and end-of-life issues. The site has an online bookstore and a search engine for finding information on end-of-life subjects. The Growth House hosts the Inter-Institutions Collaborating Network on End-of-Life Care. This website, which has 1,500 pages, has a link to the WIT Film Project.

Hospice Foundation of America
www.hospicefoundation.org
2001 S Street NW, Suite 300, Washington, DC 20009
Phone: 1-800-854-3402
This foundation sponsors an annual Living with Grief teleconference series as well as a monthly bereavement newsletter and other publications. It also has information on locating a hospice and an end-of-life database for the US.

Hospice International
www.hospiceinternational.com
Hospice International is a comprehensive website that lists Canadian hospice organizations and their websites. This is the site for anyone in Canada looking for a nearby hospice. It also lists hospices worldwide, end-of-life organizations, news sources, and the websites of related organizations such as the Multiple Sclerosis Society of Canada. The site also provides information on grief and bereavement.

Last Acts
www.lastacts.org
This site is a call-to-action campaign dedicated to improve the lives of dying patients by organizing professionals and consumers interested in bringing end-of-life issues into the open. Last Acts also has an excellent bookstore specializing in books on death and dying.

Living Wills Registry Canada
www.sentex.net/~lwr/
Family physician David Williams and his wife, who live in Stratford, Ontario, established this registry in 1992. The registry's mandate is to assist people in directing their own medical treatment in the event of an incapacitating illness or injury. It discusses what a living will is and making end-of-life decisions. It also provides information on ordering a living will, an online message board, and links to useful sites.

National Hospice Organization
www.nhpco.org
1700 Diagonal Road, Suite 625, Alexandria, VA 22314
Phone: 703-837-1500 and 1-800-658-8898
NHO provides referral services to link individuals with hospices in their local communities and with various education programs.

Partnership for Caring
www.partnershipforcaring.org
1620 Eye Street, NW, Suite 202, Washington, DC 20006
Phone: 1-800-989-WILL (9455)
Partnership for Caring provides a call to action campaign designed to improve care at the end of life. Its goals are to bring end-of- life issues out into the open and to help individual and organizations pursue the search

for better ways to care for the dying. Partnership for Caring has an excellent online bookstore specializing in books on death and dying.

As the successor organization to Choice in Dying, the 1967 inventor of living wills, this non-profit organization is dedicated to fostering communication about complex end-of-life decisions. It provides advance directives, counsels patients and families, trains professionals, advocates for improved laws, and offers a range of publications and services. The website has a list of other websites on related subjects.

Wellspring
www.wellspring.ca
81 Wellesley Street East, Toronto, ON M4Y 1H6
Phone: 416- 961-1928
Wellspring has programs for individuals with a diagnosis of cancer as well as for their families and for professionals. It offers one-to-one peer support as well as support groups and coping skills programs. The Wellspring centres also provide bereavement support and short-term counselling. In Ontario there are now centres in Oakville, London, and Niagara. The website includes centre locations, information on research and additional resources.

SPECIFIC SOURCES

Caregivers

Family Caregiver Alliance
www.caregiver.org
690 Market Street, Suite 600, San Francisco, CA 94104
Phone: 415-434-3388
Founded in 1977, Family Caregiver Alliance was the first community-based, nonprofit organization in the US to address the needs of families and friends who are providing long-term care. The Alliance developed services, advocated for public and private support, conducted research, and educated the public. It now serves all the state of California and has developed an array of services and a dedicated approach to working with families based on consumer needs. Its core services include specialized information and assistance, consultation on long term care planning, services linkage and arrangement, legal and financial consultation, respite services, and counselling and education.

In Loving Memory
http://inlovingmemoryonline.org
1416 Green Run Lane, Reston, VA 20190
Phone: 703-435-3111
In Loving Memory offers mutual support, friendship, and help to parents who have lost a child.

International THEOS Foundation
322 Blvd. of the Allies, Suite 105, Pittsburgh, PA 15222
Phone: 412-471-7779
They Help Each Other Spiritually (THEOS) helps people whose spouses have died by providing educational materials and emotional support for the newly widowed.

Tragedy Assistance Program For Survivors
www.taps.org
2001 S Street, NW, Suite 300, Washington, DC 20009
Phone: 1-800-959-TAPS (8277)
TAPS provides services, 24 hours each day, to those who have lost a loved one in the line of military duty, through peer support, crisis intervention, caseworkers, and grief counselling referrals.

Children and Death and Dying

Candlelighters Childhood Cancer Foundation
www.candlelighters.org
P.O. Box 498, Kensington, MD 20895
Phone: 301-962-3520 or 1-800-366-2223
The Candlelighters Foundation provides support and information about childhood cancer to families with children who have cancer, professionals, and adult survivors of childhood cancer. The organization has local chapters with support groups. This website has a section for kids, teens, and siblings.

Children's Hospice International
www.chionline.org
901 North Pitt Street, Suite 230, Alexandria, VA 22314
Phone: 703-684-0330 or 1-800-2-4-CHILD
The Hospice provides medical and technical assistance, research, and education for children with life-threatening conditions and their fami-

lies. The site includes information on how to tell children that they have a life-threatening illness and sections designed for children.

The Dougy Center
www.dougy.org or www.grievingchild.org
3909 S.E. 52nd Avenue, Portland, OR 97206
Phone: 503-775-5683
The Center provides age-specific (3–5, 6–12, and teens) and loss-specific (parent death, sibling death, survivors of homicide/violent death, survivors of suicide) support groups for grieving children. The Center also provides consultations to schools. It has locations in Canada and the United Kingdom.

Kids Help Phone
http://kidshelp.sympatico.ca
National Office, 300-439 University Avenue, Toronto, ON M5G 1Y8
Phone: 416-586-5437 and 1-800-668-6868
Kids Help Phone is a free, bilingual, 24-hour telephone counselling service for children and youth. Children can talk about anything, including suicide, death, school, parents, drugs, violence, and sex. Professional counsellors staff the service and offer callers counselling or refer them to services in their own community.

The Never-Ending Squirrel Tale
www.squirreltales.com
P.O. Box 1562 Columbia, MD 21044-0562
Parents of kids with cancer write this website, which offers practical tips and encouragement. This site has information about Canadian and American resources.

Diseases

AIDS
Canadian AIDS Society
www.cdnaids.ca
309 Cooper Street, 4th Floor, Ottawa, ON K2P 0G5
Phone: 613-230-3580
The Canadian AIDS Society is a coalition of 115 community based AIDS organizations across Canada. Its goal is to strengthen the response to AIDS and to enrich the lives of people and communities living with

AIDS. The website discusses resources, offers a member's section, and lists events, contacts, and related links. It also has a search engine.

Canadian AIDS Treatment Information Exchange (CATIE)
www.catie.ca
555 Richmond Street West, Suite 505, Box 1104, Toronto, ON M5V 3B1
Phone: 416-203-7122 or 1-800-263-1638
CATIE offers medical information resources to people who wish to manage their own health care in partnership with their physicians. The website also lists related websites one can access.

Critical Path AIDS Project
critpath.org/cpap/index.php
The AIDS Library (one of several programs)
1233 Locust Street, 2nd Floor, Philadelphia, PA 19107
Phone: 215-985-4851
Critical Path runs projects related to education and prevention of HIV/ AIDS. The Library answers questions by phone, fax, or email. This website, which has links to other HIV groups, discusses treatment and research, treatment and benefits, activist resources, and action alerts. It also links to Philadelphia Fight, an HIV organization.

The Hopkins HIV Report
www.hopkins-AIDS.edu
Richard W. Dunning, MHS, managing editor, Hopkins HIV Report
2700 Light House Point, Suite 220, Baltimore, MD 21224
Phone: 410-502-7907
The Hopkins HIV Report is a bimonthly newsletter for practitioners caring for patients with HIV/AIDS. Faculty from the Schools of Medicine, Public Health, and Nursing at the Johns Hopkins AIDS Service write all the articles. John Bartlett, chief of the division has published two books: *The Medical Management of HIV* (co-authored by Dr Joel Gallant) and *The Guide to Living with HIV Infection.*

International Association of Physicians in AIDS Care
www.iapac.org
33 North LaSalle Street, Suite 1700, Chicago, IL 60602-2601
Phone: 312-795-4930

This site features treatment news and clinical trial highlights, as well as information on conferences, public policy, medical education, and prevention. It lists international treatment guidelines and IAPAC publications. The website has a section on palliative care.

The HIV Daily Briefing
www.aegis.com
P.O. Box 184, San Juan Capistrano, CA 92693-0184
Phone: 949-248-5843
The HIV Daily Briefing updates worldwide AIDS/HIV news from AIDS Education Global Information Systems (AEGIS).

Gay Men's Health Crisis (GMHC)
www.gmhc.org
The Tisch Building, 119 W 24th Street. New York, NY 10011
Phone: 212-807-6655, AIDS Hotline: 1-800-243-7692
America's oldest and largest AIDS service organization, GMHC offers a variety of services, including legal assistance, nutrition counselling, family services, and crisis intervention.

Names Project – Canada
www.quilt.ca
The Canadian AIDS Memorial Quilt, National Office,
2419 Davison Street Halifax, NS B3K 4K9
Phone: 902-454-5158
The Canadian AIDS Memorial Quilt has 70 sections, each composed of quilts that use pictures and words to represent the life of a person who has died of AIDS or an AIDS related illness. Each section is meant to stand on its own. The Names Project-Canada Website allows one to view all the sections of the quilt on the web.

National Association of People with AIDS
www.napwa.org
1413 K St. NW, 7th Floor, Washington, DC 20005
Phone: 202-898-0414
NAPWA provides free publications on treatment and has an extensive information and referral department that includes a fax-on-demand system. The Association also has a health and treatment department,

which provides up to date treatment information and a free bi-monthly publication, *Medical Alert* (in English and Spanish).

ARTHRITIS
The Arthritis Society
www.arthritis.ca
393 University Avenue, Suite 1700, Toronto, ON M5G 1E6
Phone: 416-979-7228
The Arthritis Society provides a variety of treatment and educational programs for people with arthritis. The website has information on these programs, including the arthritis self-management program, a news section and an "Ask an Expert" feature, as well as other internet resources.

CANCER
American Brain Tumor Association
www.abta.org
2720 River Road, Suite 146, Des Plaines, IL 60018
Phone: 847-827-9910, Patient Line: 1-800-886-2282
This not-for-profit organization offers publications dealing with brain tumors, their treatment, and ways to cope with the disease. The Association, which serves Canadians and Americans, also maintains a nation-wide listing of support groups.

American Cancer Society
www.cancer.org
1599 Clifton Road NE, Atlanta, GA 30329-4251
Phone: 1-800-ACS-2345 (24-hour line)
This nationwide, community-based, volunteer health organization is dedicated to eliminating cancer as a major health problem. The website is comprehensive and covers most types of cancers. The phone number allows access to an international list of cancer organizations.

Canadian Cancer Society
www.cancer.ca
National Office, 10 Alcorn Avenue, Suite 200,Toronto, ON M4V 3B1
Phone: 416-961-7223
The Canadian Cancer Society works actively to prevent and cure cancer. It works in the areas of research, advocacy, prevention and information. It also provides support information for individuals with cancer,

and their caregivers and friends. It has support groups and provides for practical concerns such as transportation to cancer treatment.

CancerBACUP
www.cancerbacup.org.uk
3 Bath Place, Rivington Street,
London, England EC2A 3JR
Phone: +44 (0)20 7696 9003
This is the United Kingdom's leading cancer information service. The organization has cancer information, a cancer support service, and special programs for blacks and ethnic minorities. The organization also provides information on clinical trials.

Cancer Care
www.cancercare.org
275 7th Ave, New York, NY 10001
Phone: 1-800-813-4673 (HOPE)
Cancer Care is a national organization providing comprehensive support information for patients with cancer and for their families and caregivers. Its services include a toll free counselling line offering one-to-one over-the-phone counselling and referrals to services in the local area. The site offers material on end-of-life issues, financial assistance program lists, and links to related sites. Spanish language services are available.

CA: A Cancer Journal for Clinicians Online
www.cancer.org/docroot/PUB/content/PUB_3_3_ca.asp
CA is a peer-reviewed journal published by the American Cancer Society that provides primary care physicians with up-to-date information on all aspects of cancer diagnosis, treatment, and prevention, as well as ACS-related programs and meetings. The complete text is available. Free CME is available on line.

Cancer 411.org
http://cancer411.com
15303 Ventura Blvd., Sherman Oaks, CA 91403
Phone: 1-877-CANCR41
This site is a combination of the Rory Foundation and the Joyce Foundation. The goal of Cancer 411 is to enable cancer patients, their families, and doctors to find the critical information they need as soon as

possible. The website lists clinical trials, resources, and web casts. It lists most cancers and is comprehensive and easy to use.

Chronic Lymphocytic Leukemia from GrannyBarb
and Art's Leukemia Links
www.acor.org/leukemia/storydir/barb.html
Provides links to resources and survivors' stories about CLL. It also has a CLL online support group and information about neutropenic diets.

Chronic Lymphocytic Leukemia Education Network
www.healthtalk.com/chroniclymphocyticleukemia/index.cfm
100 4th Avenue North, Suite 460, Seattle, WA 89104
Phone: 206-352-4066
Connects patients to medical experts and other people with the disease. It also provides support, information, question-and-answers, and a free newsletter.

CURE Magazine
www.curetoday.com
Cancer Information Group, LP,
3535 Worth Street, Collins Tower, Suite 185,Dallas, TX 75246
Phone: 1-800-210-CURE
CURE Magazine's goal is to bring those with cancer and their caregivers the latest cancer updates, research, and education. It has articles written by patients and special articles for caregivers.

Gilda's Club
www.gildasclub.org
322 Eight Avenue, Suite 1402, New York, NY 10001
Phone: 1-888-Gilda-4-U
This psychological support community for people with cancer and their families and friends offers support, meditation, and networking groups, potluck suppers, and social events. The Club also offers special programs for children whose parents or family members have cancer or who have cancer themselves. There are ten affiliates across the US.

Gilda Radner Familial Ovarian Cancer Registry
www.ovariancancer.com
Roswell Park Cancer Institute

Elman and Carlton Streets, Buffalo, NY 14263
Phone: 1800-OVARIAN
The Registry tracks families with a history of ovarian cancer and does research into the causes of familial ovarian cancer in collaboration with scientists at Roswell Park Cancer Institute, Stanford School of Medicine, and Cambridge University. Women who are at high risk for ovarian cancer can call the telephone hotline where volunteers provide facts and emotional and personal support. Education and peer support are also available through the hotline.

Leukemia and Lymphoma Society of America
www.leukemia.org
1311 Mamaroneck Ave., White Plains, NY 10605
Phone: 914-949-5213
The Society is dedicated to the cure of leukemia and its related cancers – lymphoma, multiple myeloma, and Hodgkin's Disease – and to improving the quality of life of patients and their families.

The Myeloproliferative Disorders
www.acor.org/diseases/hematology/mpd/
MPD Foundation #273, 858 Armitage St., Chicago, IL 60614
Phone: 773-933-7050
The site provides information on Polycythemia Vera (PV), Essential Thrombocythemia (ET), Myelofibrosis (MF), Myelodysplastic Syndrome (MDS), and Chronic Myelocytic Leukemia (CML). It also has an online support group and lists other support groups of interest.

National Brain Tumor Foundation
www.braintumor.org
22 Battery St., Suite 612, San Francisco, CA 94111-5520
Phone 415-834-9970, Information Line: 1-800-934-CURE
The Foundation provides a variety of support education, including booklets, newsletters, support group listings, assistance starting new groups, and toll-free tumour information for patients and their families. The website also includes an interactive tour of the brain.

National Cancer Institute
www.cancer.gov/newsletter
NCI Public Inquiries Office

Suite 3036A, 6116 Executive Blvd. MSC 8322, Bethesda, MD 20892-8322
Phone: 1-800-4-CANCER and 1-800-422-6237
The NCI is the largest component of the National Institutes of Health. It coordinates a national research program on cancer cause and prevention, detection and diagnosis, and treatment. In addition it provides information about cancer to patients, the public at large, and health professionals.

National Ovarian Cancer Association
www.ovariancanada.org
27 Park Road, Toronto, ON M4W 2N2
Phone: 1-877-413-7970
The Association aims to support women living with the disease, raise awareness among health care professionals and the public, and fund research to find early detection methods and improved treatments.

National Ovarian Cancer Coalition
www.ovarian.org
500 N.E. Spanish River Blvd., Suite 8, Boca Raton, FL 33431
Phone: 561-393-0005 or 1-888-OVARIAN
Goals include providing the medical community and the public with a national resource focused on ovarian cancer and providing complete information on this disease.

OncoLink
http://oncolink.upenn.edu
Abraham Cancer Center of the University of Pennsylvania
3400 Spruce Street – 2 Donner, Philadelphia, PA 19104-4283
The University of Pennsylvania Cancer Center provides clinical trial information on specific types of cancer, complete reports on the recent American Society of Clinical Oncology (ASCO) conference, as well as an archive of several conference-based, disease specific, supportive care and news-related videos.

Society of Gynecologic Oncologists of Canada
www.g-o-c.org
National Coordinator, 780 Promenade Echo Drive, Ottawa, ON K1S 5R7
Phone: 613-730-4192, x250 or 1-800-561-2416

This website includes links to Canadian cancer websites, clinical trials, and clinical practice guidelines, as well as continuing education events.

Society of Gynecologic Oncologists
www.sgo.org
401 North Michigan Ave., Chicago, IL 60611
Phone: 312-644-6610
This is the leading organization of gynecologic oncologists in the US. It aims to encourage research and raise standards of practice in preventing and treating gynecologic cancers.

"Wit" Film Project Website
www.growthhouse.org/witfilmproject
Phone: 310-478-3711 Ext. 48353
The "Wit" Film Project is an innovative medical training program that uses the Emmy Award-winning HBO film adaptation of the play *Wit* to advance education on end-of-life issues. The patient in *Wit*, who has terminal ovarian cancer and whose physicians do not address her needs, is in an experimental clinical trial. The training program, which is available to Canadian and American medical schools, allows trainees unique opportunities to learn about the technical and humanistic aspects of caring for dying patients.

Women's Cancer Network
www.wcn.org
320 W Monroe, Suite 2528, Chicago, IL 60606
This is an interactive website aimed at informing women about gynecologic cancer. Information about risk assessment, survivors, and clinical trials make this a valuable site.

DEMENTIA
Alzheimer's Association
www.alz.org
255 N. Michigan Ave., Suite 1700, Chicago, IL 60601-7633
Phone: 312-335-8700 and 1-800-272-3900
This association provides caregiver resources and information on current medical research and public policy. It is the only national voluntary organization in the US dedicated to curing Alzheimer's disease and

providing education and support to people with the disease and their caregivers. The Association provides referrals to local chapters and support groups.

Alzheimer Society of Canada
www.alzheimer.ca
20 Eglington Ave. W., Suite 1200, Toronto, ON M4R 1K8
Phone: 416-488-8772 and 1-800-616-8816 (for use in Canada)
This Society's website offers information on treatment and research for people with Alzheimer's disease, their caregivers, and health professionals. There is an online support section, a section titled "I have Alzheimer's disease," a creative space, and a physician's corner.

DIABETES
Canadian Diabetes Association
www.diabetes.ca
National Life Building, 1400–522 University Ave., Toronto, ON M5G 2R5
Phone: 1-800-226-8464 or 416-363-0177
The goal of this organization is to provide service to Canadians affected with diabetes in a knowledgeable, respectful, and proactive way. The website provides information on consumer literature on diabetes, information sessions and forums, resource centres, insurance issues, summer camps, peer-support groups, cooking programs, and grocery store tours.

DIGESTIVE DISEASES
American Liver Foundation
www.liverfoundation.org
75 Maiden Lane, Suite 603, New York, NY 10038
Phone: 1-800-GOLIVER (465-4837)
This national non-profit organization is dedicated to preventing, treating, and conquering hepatitis and other diseases of the liver and gallbladder. The website has general information on liver health and clinical trials.

HEART DISEASE
American Heart Association
www.americanheart.org
7272 Greenville Avenue, Dallas, TX 75231
Phone: 214-373-6300 or 1-800-242-8721 (for a connection to the closest affiliate)

The Association is committed to reducing disability and death from cardiovascular diseases and stroke.

Heart and Stroke Foundation of Canada
www.heartandstroke.ca
222 Queen Street, Suite 1402 Ottawa, ON K1P 5V9
Phone: 613-569-4361
This organization's goals are to improve the health of Canadians by preventing and reducing disability and death from heart disease and stroke through research, health promotion, and advocacy. The website has information on healthy eating (including recipes) and on heart disease, stroke, and local events. It also discusses the goals of research, health promotion, and volunteering at length and offers a personal health assessment tool.

KIDNEY DISEASES
National Kidney Foundation
www.kidney.org
30 East 33rd Street, Suite 1100, New York, NY 10016
Phone: 1-800-622-9010 or 212-889-2210
The Foundation supports research projects and sponsors community programs in treatment, service, education, and prevention of diseases of the kidney and urinary tract.

NEUROLOGICAL DISEASES
ALS Society of Canada
www.als.ca
265 Yorkland Blvd, Suite 300, Toronto, ON M2J 1S5
Phone: 1-800-267-4257
The goal of the ALS Society is to support research towards a cure for Amyotrophic Lateral Sclerosis (ALS), commonly referred to as Lou Gehrig's disease, and to support ALS partners in the provision of quality care for all persons affected by ALS. The website has recent news and articles with information on ALS and recent research news. It also lists ALS events and clinics across Canada.

ALS Association of the USA
www.alsa.org
27001 Agoura Road, Suite 150, Calabasas Hills, CA 91301
Phone: 1-818-880-9007

This is America's national information resource for Amyotrophic Lateral Sclerosis (ALS), commonly known as Lou Gehrig's disease.

American Parkinson Disease Association
http://apdaparkinson.com
1250 Hylan Blvd., Suite 4B, Staten Island, NY 10305
Phone 1-888-223-2732
The Association is committed to serving the Parkinson community through a comprehensive program of research, education, and support.

Multiple Sclerosis Society of Canada
www.mssociety.ca
175 Bloor Street East, Suite 700, North Tower, Toronto, ON M4W 3R8
Phone: 416-922-6065 or 1-800-268-7582
The Multiple Sclerosis Society of Canada advocates and provides support for individuals with multiple sclerosis (MS) and raises money for MS research. The website has general information on MS and MS research. It also lists information on community activities and provides other useful information.

National Institute of Neurological Disorders and Stroke (NINDS)
www.ninds.nih.gov
NIH Neurological Institute, P.O. Box 5801, Bethesda, MD 20824
Phone: 301-496-5751 or 1-800-352-9424
The website for this division of the NIH provides general science-based information about selected neurological disorders, NINDS-funded clinical trials and clinical studies (including those on chronic pain research), and clinical advisories and alerts.

National Multiple Sclerosis Society of the USA
www.nationalmssociety.org
7333 Third Avenue, New York, NY 10017
Phone: 1-800-FIGHT MS or 212-476-0436
This is a comprehensive worldwide resource on MS-related information, offering more than 2,000 support groups to aid families in dealing with the challenges of chronic illness. (MS is not a terminal illness except in the rarest cases.)

National Parkinson Foundation
www.parkinson.org

1501 NW 9th Ave, Bob Hope Road
Miami, FL 33136-1494
Phone: 1-800-327-4545 or 305-547-6666
The Foundation is committed to finding the cause and cure for Parkinson's disease and other allied neurological disorders through research, providing diagnostic and therapeutic services, improving the quality of life for patients and caregivers, and educating people about Parkinson's disease. This site lists centres of excellence in Canada.

National Stroke Association
www.stroke.org
9707 E. Easter Lane, Englewood, CO 80112-5112
Phone 303-649-9299 or 1-800-STROKES or 1-800-787-6537
The Association is dedicated to the prevention, treatment, and research of stroke, and to the support of stroke victims and their caregivers.

NeuroGenetic Surgery:
Neurosurgery at Massachusetts General Hospital/Harvard
http://neurosurgery.mgh.harvard.edu/NeuroGeneticSurgery
Director, MGH Neurogenetics Unit, Wang ACC-835
Massachusetts General Hospital
Boston, MA 02114
Phone: 617-726-5732
The Massachusetts General Hospital/Harvard Medical School site includes links to the NeuroGenetics Center, NeuroGenetic Clinic, and NeuroFibromatosis Clinic. The NeuroGenetics Center facilitates surgical and non-surgical multidisciplinary management of inherited neurological syndromes. Each area includes an index of links to information and research and to lists of MGH neurosurgeons with expertise in neurogenetic disorders. A physician may request a second opinion by faxing a brief medical history to this website.

NeuroNet
www.neuro-net.net
NeuroNet's content is organized under dementia, acute stroke, epilepsy, and multiple sclerosis. Access to NeuroNet is limited to physicians and requires pre-registration. Once registered, physicians may access news from *The Chronicle of Neurology & Psychiatry*, participate in physician-only forums, and find links to information on congresses and medical education. The site also has free continuing medical education (CME).

PULMONARY DISEASES
American Lung Association
www.lungusa.org
61 Broadway, 6th Floor
New York, NY 10006
Phone: 212-315-8700
The Association is dedicated to preventing lung disease, with a nation-wide priority on asthma.

Cystic Fibrosis Foundation
www.cff.org
6931 Arlington Road
Bethesda, MD 20814
Phone: 1-800-344-4823 or 301-951-4422
The Foundation is dedicated to the development of means to cure and control cystic fibrosis (CF) and to the improvement of the quality of life of those with the disease.

The Lung Association National Office for Canada
www.lung.ca/ca
3 Raymond Street, Suite 300
Ottawa, ON K1R 1A3
Phone: 613-569-6411
The goals of the Lung Association are to help all Canadians to enjoy clean air and to have healthy lungs. The website includes information on living with lung diseases, including asthma, chronic lung disease, sleep apnea, tuberculosis, as well as many other lung diseases. It has information on the respiratory system in general, on air quality, smoking, tobacco, research, and a special children's corner.

Pulmonary Fibrosis Foundation
www.pulmonaryfibrosis.org
1440 West Washington Blvd.
Chicago, IL 60607
Phone: 312-277-6895
The Foundation's goal is to find a cure by supporting research into new treatments, including stem cell research implants for stimulating new lung cell growth. They also aim to advance the education of physicians to improve the early diagnosis of this serious disease. Information about clinical trials is available.

SLEEP DISORDERS
Canadian Sleep Society
www.css.to
School of Psychology, Laval University
Sainte-Foy, QC G1K 7P4
This is a professional association of clinicians, scientists, and technologists whose goal is to advance research and education about sleep disorders. The website lists links to sleep journals and has information about sleep disorders.

National Institute of Health, National Center for Sleep Disorders Research
www.nhlbi.nih.gov/sleep/
National Heart, Lung, and Blood Institute Health Information Center
P.O. Box 30105
Betheseda, MD 20824-0105
Phone: 301-592-8573
The agency coordinates and provides information to government supported sleep research, training, and education to improve the health of Americans. It produces pamphlets on sleep that can be downloaded to the computer; it also has online interactive questionnaires and information on other sleep agencies.

National Sleep Foundation
www.sleepfoundation.org
1522 K.Street NW, Suite 500
Washington, DC 2005
Phone: 202-347-3471
The National Sleep Foundation is a nonprofit organization that seeks to improve public health and safety by achieving an understanding of sleep and sleep disorders and by supporting sleep related education, research, and advocacy.

Medical Organizations

American Academy of Hospice & Palliative Medicine
www.aahpm.org
4700 West Lake Avenue, Glenview, IL 60025-1485
Phone: 847-375-4712
This international organization of physicians is dedicated to the advancement of palliative medicine in the management of patients

with terminal illness. The site includes information on certification in Hospice and Palliative Medicine administered by the American Board of Hospice and Palliative Medicine.

American Medical Association
www.ama-assn.org
515 N. State Street, Chicago, IL 60610
Phone: 312-464-5000 or 1-800-621-8335
The AMA's website contains extensive links to disease- and condition-related sites on the World Wide Web.

American Nurses Association
www.nursingworld.org
600 Maryland Ave. SW, Suite 100 West,
Washington, DC 20024-2571
Phone: 1-800-274-4ANA
This is the largest professional organization representing registered nurses in the US.

American Osteopathic Association
www.aoa-net.org or www.osteopathic.org
Phone: 1-800-621-1773 or 312-202-8000
The site has consumer health information on a wide variety of topics, including end-of-life care.

Association for Death Education & Counseling
www.adec.org
342 North Main Street, West Hartford, CT 06117-2507
Phone: 860-586-7503
ADEC is dedicated to improving the quality of death education and death-related counselling and care giving. This site has an excellent list of related websites.

Association of Pediatric Oncology Nurses
www.apon.org
4700 W. Lake Ave.
Glenview, IL 60025
Phone: 847-375-4724
This is the professional organization for pediatric oncology nurses and other pediatric health care professionals specializing in hematology/

oncology. The chief focus is on promoting the best nursing care for children and adolescents with cancer.

Canadian Medical Association
www.cma.ca/cma
1867 Alta Vista Drive
Ottawa, ON K1G 3Y6
Phone: 1-800-457-4205
CMA is the voice of Canadian physicians. It acts as an advocate for patient access to high-quality health care and provides leadership and guidance to physicians. The CMA publishes six specialty journals. The website also has a student section.

Canadian Nurses Association
www.cna-nurses.ca
50 Driveway
Ottawa, ON K2P 1E2
Phone: 613-237-2133 or 1-800-361-8404
The Canadian Nurses Association is a federation of 11 provincial and territorial nursing associations, representing more than 116,000 registered nurses. This website has links to specialty nursing groups.

Health Canada
www.hc-sc.gc.ca
A.L. 0900C2
Ottawa, ON K1A 0K9
Phone: 613-957-2991
Health Canada is the federal department responsible for helping people in Canada maintain and improve their health. It administers the Canada Health Act. The website has information on healthy living, diseases, and health promotion. It has a section dedicated to children who have cancer and a section for individuals with AIDS. Both sections discuss end-of-life issues, including dying at home.

Mental Health Organizations

The Canadian Mental Health Association
www.cmha.ca
8 King Street East, Suite 810, Toronto, ON M5C 1B5
Phone: 416-484-7750

The Canadian Mental Health Association provides direct services to over 100,000 Canadians yearly. The Association's tools include information services, sponsored research projects, seminars, pamphlets, newsletters, and research centres. The website has an article called "Grieving," which discusses the stages of grieving, how to help a friend who is grieving, how to cope with one's grief, and where to get more help in Canada. There is also an article on suicide.

Suicide Information and Education Centre
www.siec.ca
Suite 320, 1202 Centre Street S.E., Calgary, AB T2G 5A5
Phone: 403-245-3900
The Centre is a special library and resource centre that provides information on suicide and suicidal behavior. It also conducts training programs for caregivers on intervention, awareness, bereavement and crisis management. (It is not a crisis hot line.)

Other Professional Organizations

ETHICS
The Bioethics Education Project
http://eduserv.hscer.washington.edu/bioethics
c/o The Department of Medical History and Ethics, Box 357120
University of Washington School of Medicine, Seattle, WA 98195
Bioethics topics, such as advance care planning, breaking bad news, do-not-resuscitate orders, difficult patients, termination of life-sustaining treatment, and truth-telling and withholding information, are discussed with case-based scenarios linked to each topic. The Project also presents recommended readings in a question and answer format.

University of Toronto Joint Centre for Bioethics
www.utoronto.ca/jcb/
88 College Street, Toronto, ON M5G 1L4
Phone: 416-978-2709
The Centre "includes a clinical ethics group that seeks to develop models of clinical ethics practice in diverse health care settings. The group does consultation, teaching, organizational/clinical initiatives, research, and community outreach."

PAIN, PALLIATIVE CARE, AND CRITICAL CARE
American Academy of Pain Management
www.aapainmanage.org
13947 Mono Way #A.
Sonora, CA 95370
Phone: 209-533-9744
This website can help patients find a qualified pain professional in all areas of the US. Continuing education and pain specialty accreditation is also available through this site. Clinical conferences are organized on an annual basis.

Beth Israel Medical Center Department of Pain Medicine & Palliative Care
www.stoppain.org
First Avenue at 16th Street
New York, NY 10003
Phone: 877-620-9999
This site discusses pain, pain clinical trials, and has resources for patients and professionals. It also addresses end-of-life care, hospice, and ethical and legal issues in palliative care. Online conferences are available.

Medical College of Wisconsin – Palliative Care Center
www.mcw.edu/pallmed
8701 Watertown Plank Rd.
Milwaukee, WI 53226
Phone: 414-456-8296
"The Palliative Care Center is committed to improving care for the dying in America through the development, implementation and dissemination of innovative education and clinical care programs." The Program has educational, research, and patient care components. This website lists related sites.

University of Wisconsin Pain and Policy Studies Group
www.medsch.wisc.edu/painpolicy
University of Wisconsin Medical School,
Pain and Policy Studies Group
406 Science Drive, Suite 202
Madison, WI 53711-1068
Phone: 608-263-7662

The primary concern of this group is adequate pain management for patients in severe pain. The Group is interested in studying public policy in order to identify possible barriers to the medical use of available analgesics.

Society of Critical Care Medicine
www.sccm.org
701 Lee Street, Suite 200
Des Plaines, IL 60016
Phone: 847-827-6869

This site is designed for anyone who seeks information on critical care medicine. Critical care combines the efforts of physicians, nurses, respiratory therapists, pharmacists, pharmacologists, and allied health professionals in the coordinated and collaborative management of patients with life-threatening illness and single or multiple organ system failure. Critical care is most often practised in the ICU.

References

ABBREVIATIONS

Acad. Med.	*Academic Medicine*
Acta Psychiatr. Scand.	*Acta Psychiatrica Scandinavica*
Alcohol Health Res. World	*Alcohol Health and Research World*
Am. Fam. Physician	*American Family Physician*
Am. J. Epidemiology	*American Journal of Epidemiology*
Am. J. Hosp. Palliat. Care	*The American Journal of Hospice and Palliative Care*
Am. J. Med.	*The American Journal of Medicine*
Am. J. Psychiatry	*The American Journal of Psychiatry*
Am. Med. News	*American Medical News*
Ann. Emerg. Med.	*Annals of Emergency Medicine*
Ann. Intern. Med.	*Annals of Internal Medicine*
Ann. N.Y. Acad. Sci.	*Annals of the New York Academy of Sciences*
Arch. Dis. Child.	*Archives of Disease in Childhood*
Arch. Intern. Med.	*Archives of Internal Medicine*
Arch. Gen. Psychiatry	*Archives of General Psychiatry*
Beh. Res. Ther	*Behavior Research and Therapy*
BMJ	*British Medical Journal*
Br. J. Psychiatry	*British Journal of Psychiatry*
Cancer Causes Control	*Cancer Causes and Control: CCC*
Can. Fam. Physician	*Canadian Family Physician*
Can. J. Psychiatry	*Canadian Journal of Psychiatry*
Can. Med. Assoc. J.	*Canadian Medical Association Journal*
Clin. Geriatr. Med.	*Clinics in Geriatrics Medicine*
Crit. Care Med.	*Critical Care Medicine*
Death Stud	*Death Studies*

Emerg. Med. Clin. North Am.	*Emergency Medicine Clinics of North America*
Fam. Pract.	*Family Practice*
J. Affect. Disord.	*Journal of Affective Disorders*
J. Am. Coll. Cardiol.	*Journal of the American College of Cardiology*
J. Am. Geriatr. Soc.	*Journal of American Geriatrics Society*
J. Adv. Nurs.	*Journal of Advanced Nursing*
J. Clin. Epidemiol.	*Journal of Clinical Epidemiology*
J. Clin. Oncol.	*Journal of Clinical Oncology*
J. Chronic Dis.	*Journal of Chronic Diseases*
J. Clin. Ethics	*The Journal of Clinical Ethics*
J. Consult. Clin. Psychol.	*Journal of Consulting and Clinical Psychology*
J. Drug Ed.	*Journal of Drug Education*
J. Emerg. Med.	*The Journal of Emergency Medicine*
J. Fam. Pract.	*The Journal of Family Practise*
J. Gen. Intern. Med.	*Journal of General Internal Medicine*
J. Law Med. Ethics	*The Journal of Law, Medicine, and Ethics*
J. Leg. Med.	*The Journal of Legal Medicine*
J. Neurol.	*Journal of Neurology*
J. Pain Symptom Manag.	*Journal of Pain and Symptom Management*
J. Prof. Nurs.	*Journal of Professional Nursing*
J. Reprod. Med.	*The Journal of Reproductive Medicine*
JAMA	*Journal of the American Medical Association*
Jt. Comm. J. Qual. Improv.	*The Joint Commission Journal on Quality Improvement*
N. Engl. J. Med.	*The New England Journal of Medicine*
NHO Newsline	*National Hospice Organization Newsline*
Occup. Med.	*Occupational Medicine*
Palliat. Med.	*Palliative Medicine*
Postgrad. Med.	*Postgraduate Medicine*
Qual. Life Res.	*Quality of Life Research: An International Journal*
Scand. J. Prim. Health Care	*Scandinavian Journal of Primary Health Care*
West J. Med.	*The Western Journal of Medicine*

a'Brook, M. 1990. "Psychosis and depression." *The Practitioner* 234: 992–3.

Adam, J. 1997. "ABC of palliative care. The last 48 hours." *BMJ* 315: 1600–3.

Adams, D. 2003. "Peer pressure." *Am. Med. News* 46: 9–10.

Alcoholics Anonymous. 2001. *The Big Book.* (4th ed.) New York: Alcoholics Anonymous World Services, Inc.

Alexander, D.A. 1998. "Psychosocial research in palliative care." In D. Doyle, G.W.C. Hanks, and N. MacDonald, eds., *Oxford Textbook of Palliative Medicine.* (2nd ed.) Oxford: Oxford University Press.

Allebeck, P., C. Bolund, and G. Ringback. 1989. "Increased suicide rate in cancer patients: A cohort study based on the Swedish Cancer Register." *J. Clin. Epidemiol.* 42:611–16.

American Board of Internal Medicine. 1996. *Caring for the Dying: Identification and Promotion of Physician Competency.* Philadelphia: American Board of Internal Medicine.

The American College Dictionary. 1966. New York: Random House.

American Society of Clinical Oncology. 1998. "Cancer care during the last phase of life." *J. Clin. Oncol.* 16, 5: 1986–96.

Arnetz, B.B., L.G. Horte, A. Hedberg, et al. 1987. "Suicide patterns among physicians related to other academics as well as to the general population; Results from a national long term prospective study." *Acta Psychiatr. Scand.* 75, 2: 139–43.

Ascher, L.M., R. Turner. 1979. "Paradoxical intention and insomnia: An experimental investigation." *Behav. Res. Ther.* 17, 4: 408–11.

Balk, D.E. 1993. "Sibling death, adolescent bereavement, and religion." *Death Stud.* 15:1–20.

Balor, T.F., and M. Grant. 1989. "From clinical research to secondary prevention: International collaboration in the development of the Alcohol Use Disorders Identification Test (AUDIT)." *Alcohol Health Res. World.* 13: 371–4.

Barroso, P., E. Osuna, and A. Luna. 1992. "Doctors' death experience and attitudes towards death, euthanasia, and informing terminal patients." *Medicine and Law* 11: 527–33.

Bedell, S.E., K. Cadenhead, and T.B. Graboys. 2001. "The doctor's letter of condolence." *N. Engl. J. Med.* 344, 15: 1162–4.

Berger, J. 1967. *A Fortunate Man: The Story of A Country Doctor.* New York: Random House.

Berman, S. 1997. "The quality of dying: How can we improve care at the end of life." *Jt. Comm. J. Qual. Improv.* 23, 9: 498–504.

Black, D., et al. 1989. "Educating medical students about death and dying." *Arch. Dis. Child.* 64: 750–3.

Blackburn, I.M., S. Bishop, et al. 1981. "The efficacy of cognitive therapy in depression: A treatment trial using cognitive therapy and pharmacotherapy, each alone and in combination." *Br. J. Psychiatry* 139: 181–9.

Blackburn I.M., and R.G. Moore. 1997. "Controlled acute and follow-up trial of cognitive therapy and pharmaco-therapy in patients with recurrent depression." *Br. J. Psychiatry* 171: 328–34.

Block, S.D. 2001. "Psychological considerations, growth, and transcendence at the end of life: The art of the possible." *JAMA* 285, 22: 2898–905.

Bluebond-Langer, M. 1978. *The Private World of Dying Children.* Princeton: Princeton University Press.

Bombeck, E. 1989. *I Want to Grow Hair, I Want to Grow Up, I Want to Go to Boise.* New York: Harper and Row.

Bootzin, R.R., M.L. Perlis. 1992. "Nonpharmacological treatments of insomnia." *Journal of Clinical Psychiatry* 53 (Supplement 6): 37–41.

Bradley, K.A., J. Boyd-Wickizer, S.H. Powell, et al. 1998. "Alcohol screening questionnaires in women." *JAMA* 280, 2: 166–7.

Breitbart, W., E. Bruera, H. Chochinov, et al. 1995. "Neuropsychiatric syndromes and psychological symptoms in patients with advanced cancer." *J. Pain Symptom Manag.* 10: 131–41.

Breitbart, W., B. Rosenfeld, H. Pessin, et al. 2000. "Depression, hopelessness, and desire for hastened death in terminally ill patients with cancer." *JAMA* 284, 22: 2907–11.

British Medical Association. 1993. *The Morbidity and Mortality of the Medical Profession.* London: British Medical Association.

Brown, R. 1996. "Treating AIDS: Hope and despair." *Can. Med. Assoc. J.* 152, 2: 139–45.

Bruera, E. 1998. "Research into symptoms other than pain." In Doyle, Hanks, and MacDonald, eds. *Oxford Textbook of Palliative Medicine.*

Buckman, R. 1988. *I Don't Know What to Say: How to Help and Support Someone Who Is Dying.* New York: Vintage Books.

– 1993. *How to Break Bad News – A Guide For Health Care Professionals.* London: Macmillan Medical.

– 1998. "Communication in palliative care: A practical guide." In Doyle, Hanks, and McDonald, eds., *Oxford Textbook of Palliative Care.*

Burns, D. 1989. *The Feeling Good Handbook.* New York: Penguin Books.

Calman, K., and G. Hanks. 1998. "Clinical and health services research." In Doyle, Hanks, and McDonald, eds., *Oxford Textbook of Palliative Care.*

Canadian Centre on Substance Abuse. 2003. "Alcohol overview." www.ccsa.ca/index.asp?page=83

Carrese, J.A., and L.A. Rhodes. 1995. "Western bioethics in the Navajo reservation: Benefit or harm?" *JAMA* 274: 826–9.

Carron, A.T., J. Lynn, and P. Keaney. 1999. "End-of-life care in medical textbooks." *Ann. Intern. Med.* 130: 82–6.

Casarett, D.J., and S.K. Inouye. 2001. "Diagnosis and management of delirium near the end of life." *Ann. Intern. Med.* 135: 32–40.

Cassidy, S. 1988. *Sharing the Darkness*. London: Darton, Longman, and Todd.

Chambers, R., and J.Belcher. 1994. "Predicting mental health problems in general practitioners." *Occup. Med.* 44, 4: 212–16.

Chochinov, H.M., K.G. Wilson, M. Ennis, et al. 1995. "Desire for death in the terminally Ill." *Am. J. Psychiatry* 152: 1185–9.

Clay, R.A. 2000. "Psychotherapy is cost-effective." *Monitor on Psychology* 31, 1: 40–1.

Coles, R. 1990. *The Spiritual Life of Children*. Boston: Houghton Mifflin Co.

Copp, G. 1998. "A review of current theories of death and dying." *J. Adv. Nurs.* 28, 2: 382–90.

Corr, C.A. 1992. "A task-based approach to coping with dying." *Omega* 24, 2: 81–4.

Corr, C.D., J.D. Morgan, and H. Wass, eds. 1993. "International Work Group on Death, Dying, and Bereavement: Statements on Death, Dying and Bereavement." London, Ontario: International Work Group on Death, Dying, and Bereavement.

Council on Scientific Affairs. 1987. "Results and implications of the AMA-APA physician mortality project: Stage II." *JAMA* 257, 2: 2949–53 [Erratum, *JAMA*, 1987, 258, 5: 614].

Cousins, N. 1979. *Anatomy of an Illness*. New York: W.W. Norton.

Covey, S. 1989. *The Seven Habits of Highly Effective People*. New York: Fireside Books.

Covinsky, K.E., J.D. Fuller, K. Yaffe, et al. 2000. "Communication and decision-making in seriously ill patients: Finding of the SUPPORT project." *J. Am. Geriatr. Soc.* 48: S187–S93.

Cruzan vs. Director, 1990. Missouri Department of Health. 497 US 261. Docket number: 88-1503.

Curtis, J.R., and D. Patrick. 1997. "Barriers to communication about end-of-life care in AIDS patients." *J. Gen. Intern. Med.* 12: 736–41.

Curtis, J.R., D.L. Patrick, et al. 2000. "Why don't patients and physicians talk about end-of-life care?" *Arch. Intern. Med.* 160: 1690–6.

Davidson, K.W., C. Hackler, D.R. Caradine, et al. 1989. "Physicians' attitudes on advance directives." *JAMA* 262: 2415–19.

Davies, E., and B. Eng. 1998. "Special issues in bereavement and staff support." In Doyle, Hanks, and McDonald, eds., *Oxford Textbook of Palliative Care*.

Dawson, S. 1995. "A Dying Child." *Can. Fam. Physician* 41: 1534–40.

de Veber, L.L. 1995. "The influence of spirituality on dying children's perception of death." In Adams, D.N. and E.J. Deveau, eds. *The Innocence of Childhood: Helping Children and Adolescents Cope with Life-Threatening Illness and Dying*. Amityville, NY: Baywood Publishing.

– 2001. Personal Communication with authors.

Ditto, P.H., W.D. Smucker, J.H. Danks, et al. 2003. "Stability of older adults' preferences for life-sustaining medical treatment." *Health Psychology* 22, 6: 605–15.

Donaldson, M.S., and M.J. Field. 1998. "Measuring quality of care at the end of life." *Arch. Intern. Med.* 158: 121–8.

Doyle, D., G.W.C. Hanks, and N. MacDonald, eds. 1998. *Oxford Textbook of Palliative Medicine.* (2nd ed.) Oxford: Oxford University Press.

Easwaran, E. 1982. *God Makes Rivers to Flow: Passages for Meditation.* Tomales, CA: Nilgiri Press.

– 1994. *Take Your Time: Finding Balance in a Hurried World.* Tomales, CA: Nilgiri Press.

Edlich, R., and E. Kübler-Ross. 1992. "On death and dying in the emergency department." *J. Emerg. Med.* 10: 225–9.

Eisenberg, M.S., and T.J. Mengert. 2001. "Cardiac resuscitation." *N. Engl. J. Med.* 344: 1304–13.

Elkin, I., M.T. Shea, J.T. Watkins, et al. 1989. "National Institute of Mental Health treatment of depression collaborative research program: General effectiveness of treatments." *Arch. Gen. Psychiatry* 46: 971–82.

Emanuel, L.L., M.J. Barry, J.D. Stoeckle, et al. 1991. "Advance directives for medical care – A case for greater use." *N. Engl. J. Med.* 324: 889–95.

Emanuel, E.J., and L.L. Emanuel. 1998. "The promise of a good death." *The Lancet* 351: 21–9.

Emanuel, L.L., C.F. von Gunten, and F.D. Ferris, eds. 1999. "Education for Physicians on End-of-Life Care." *American Medical Association.* www.EPEC.net.

Emanuel, E.J., D.L. Fairclough, and L.L. Emanuel. 2000. "Attitudes and desires related to euthanasia and physician-assisted suicide among terminally ill patients and their caregivers." *JAMA* 284, 19: 2460–8.

Espie, C.A., W.R. Lindsay, D.N. Brooks, et al. 1989. "A controlled comparative investigation of psychological treatments for chronic sleep-onset insomnia." *Behav. Res. Ther.* 27, 1: 79–88.

Faber-Langedoen, K., and P.N. Lanken, for the ACP-ASIM End-of-Life Care Consensus Panel. 2000. "Dying patients in the ICU: Forgoing treatment, maintaining care." *Ann. Intern. Med.* 133, 11: 886–93.

Fallowfield, L.J. 2002. "Truth may hurt but deceit hurts more: Communication in palliative care." *Palliat. Med.* 16: 297–303.

Fava, G.A., et al. 1998. "Prevention of recurrent depression with cognitive behavioral therapy: Preliminary findings." *Arch. Gen. Psychiatry.* 55, 9: 816–20.

Frampton, D.R. 1998. "Creative arts and literature." In Doyle, Hanks, and MacDonald, eds., *Oxford Textbook of Palliative Medicine.*

Friedman, M. 1974. *The Story of Josh.* New York: Ballantine Books.

Gabbard, G.O., and C. Nadelsen. 1995. "Professional boundaries in the physician patient relationship." *JAMA* 273, 18: 1145–59.

Gamble, E.R., P.J. McDonald, and P.R. Lichstein. 1991. "Knowledge, attitudes, and behavior of elderly persons regarding living wills." *Arch. Intern. Med.* 51: 277–80.

Garwin, M. 1998. "The duty to care – the right to refuse." *J. Leg. Med.* 19: 99–125.

Gatrad, A.R. 1994. "Muslim customs surrounding death, bereavement, postmortem examinations, and organ transplants." *BMJ* 309: 521–3.

Gazelle, G. 1998a. "The slow code." *N. Engl. J. Med.* 338: 1921–3.

– 1998b. "The slow code – Should anyone rush to its defense?" *N. Engl. J. Med.* 338: 467–9.

Geddes, J., R. Butler, and S. Hatcher. 2003. "Depressive Disorders." *Clinical Evidence* 9: 1034–57.

Gilligan, T., and T.A. Raffin. 1996. "End-of-life discussion with patients: Timing and truth telling." *Chest.* 109: 11–12.

Glaser, B.G., and A.L. Strauss. 1965. *Awareness of Patient.* New York: Aldine.

Glaser, B.G., and Strauss, A.L. 1968. *Time for Dying.* Chicago: Aldine.

Glasser, W. 1976. *Positive Addiction.* New York: Harper.

Gloaguen, V., J. Cottraux, M. Cucherat, et al. 1998. "A meta-analysis of the effects of cognitive therapy in depressed people." *J. Affect. Disord.* 49: 59–72.

Goodwin, D.W., and W.F. Gabrielli, Jr. 1997. "Alcohol: Clinical aspects." In J. H. Lowinson, P. Ruiz, R.B. Millman, and J.G. Langrod., eds., *Substance Abuse – A Comprehensive Textbook.* (3rd ed.) Baltimore: Lippincott, Williams, and Wilkins.

Gorer, G., and R.J. Kastenbaum, eds. 1979. *Death, Grief, and Mourning.* Manchester, NH: Ayer Co. Publishers.

Greer, D.S., V. Mor, J.N. Morris, et al. 1986. "An alternative in terminal care: Results of the national hospice study." *J. Chronic Dis.* 39: 9–26.

Gunther, J. 1949. *Death Be Not Proud: A Memoir.* New York: Henry Holt and Company.

Haas, J.S., J.S. Weisman, P.D. Cleary, et al. 1991. "Discussion of preferences for life-sustaining care by persons with AIDS." *Arch. Intern. Med.* 153: 1241–8.

Handler, E. 1996. *Time on Fire: My Comedy of Terrors.* New York: Henry Holt and Company.

Hanh, T.N. 1987. *Being Peace.* Berkeley, CA: Parallax Press.

– 1991. *Peace Is Every Step: The Path of Mindfulness in Everyday Life.* New York: Bantam Books.

Harper, M.B., and N. Wisian. 1994. "Care of bereaved parents: a study of patient satisfaction." *J. Reprod. Med.* 39, 2: 80–4.

Hauri, P., and S. Linde. 1990. *No More Sleepless Nights.* New York: Wiley.

Highfield, M.F. 1992. "Spiritual health of oncology patients: Nurses and patient perspectives." *Cancer Nursing.* 15, 1: 3

Hill, P.T. 1995. "Treating the dying patient: The challenge for medical education." *Arch. Intern. Med.* 155: 1265–9.

Hinton, J. 1967. *Dying.* London: Penguin.

Hsu, K., and J. Marshall. 1987. "Prevalence of depression and distress in a large sample of Canadian residents, interns, and fellows." *Am. J. Psychiatry* 144: 1561–6.

Hughes, P., et al. 1991. "Resident physician substance use in the US." *JAMA* 265: 2069–73.

Hurwitz, T.D., M. Beiser, and H. Nichol. 1987. "Impaired interns and residents." *Can. J. Psychiatry* 32: 165–9

Johnson, E.O. *Sleep in America: 1999. Results from the National Sleep Foundation's 1999 Omnibus Sleep Poll.* Washington, DC: National Sleep Foundation.

Johnson, J. 1996. "Re-examining care for the dying. AMA: Education key to making end-of-life decisions." *Amer. Med. News* 29, 48: 337–8.

James, J.W., and R. Friedman. 1998. *The Grief Recovery Handbook.* New York: Harper Collins.

Jellinek, M.S., D. Todres, E. Catlin, et al. 1993. "Pediatric intensive care training: Confronting the dark side." *Crit. Care Med.* 21, 5: 775–9

Kane, R.I., J. Wales, L. Bernstein, et al. 1984. "A randomized trial of hospice care." *The Lancet* 890–4.

Kastenbaum, R., and Kastenbaum, B. 1989. *The Encyclopedia of Death.* New York: Avon Books.

Kearl, M.C. 1989. *Ending: A Sociology of Death and Dying.* New York: Oxford University Press.

King, S.B., D.J. Ullyot, L. Basta, et al. 1998. "Task Force 2: Application of medical and surgical interventions near the end of life." *J. Am. Coll. Cardiol.* 31, 5: 933–42.

Klatsky, A.L., and M.A. Armstrong. 1992. "Alcohol, smoking, coffee, and cirrhosis." *Am. J. Epidemiol.* 36: 1248–57.

Krumholz, H.M., R.S. Phillips, M.B. Hamel et al. 1998. "Resuscitation preferences among patients with severe congestive heart failure: Results from the SUPPORT Project." *Circulation* 98 (7): 648–55.

Kübler-Ross, E. 1969. *On Death and Dying.* New York: MacMillan.

– 1978. *To Live until We Say Goodbye.* Englewood Cliffs, NJ: Prentice-Hall.

– 1983. *On Children and Death.* New York: Simon and Schuster.

La Puma, D., and R.J. Moss. 1991. "Advance directives on admission: Clinical implications and analysis of the patient self-determination act." *JAMA* 266: 402–5.

Larson, D.G., and D.R. Tobin. 2000. "End-of-life conversations." *JAMA* 284: 1573–8.

Lash, J. 1990. *The Seeker's Handbook*. New York: Harmony Books.

Lawrence, J.M. 1989. "Stress problems in the medical profession." *Australian Family Physician* 18, 11: 1379–89.

Lindeman, S., E. Laara, H. Hakko, et al. 1996. "A systematic review of gender-specific suicide mortality in medical doctors." *Br. J. Psychiatry* 168: 274–9.

Lindeman, S., E. Laara, E. Vuori, et al. 1997. "Suicides among physicians, engineers, and teachers: The prevalence of reported depression, admissions to hospital and contributory causes of death." *Acta Psychiatr. Scand.* 96: 68–71.

Listen, E.H. 1975. "Education on death and dying: A neglected area in the medical curriculum." *Omega* 6: 193–8.

Lloyd. S., D. Streiner, S. Shannon. 1994. "Burnout, depression, life, and job satisfaction among Canadian emergency physicians." *J. Emerg. Med.* 12, 4: 559–65.

Longnecker, M.P. 1994. "Alcoholic beverage consumption in relation to the risk of breast cancer: Meta-analysis and review." *Cancer Causes Control* 5: 73–82.

Lundin, T. 1984. "Morbidity following sudden and unexpected bereavement." *Br. J. Psychiatry.* 144: 84–8.

Lynn, J. 2001. "Serving patients who may die soon and their families. The role of hospice and other services." *JAMA* 285, 22: 2898–905.

Mahon, M. 1994. "Death of a sibling: Primary care interventions." *Pediatric Nursing* 20, 3: 293–8.

Mak, J.M., M. Clinton. 1999. "Promoting a good death: An agenda for outcomes research. A review of the literature." *Nursing Ethics* 6, 2: 97–106.

Malacrida, R., C.M. Bettelini, A. Degrate, et al. 1998. "Reasons for dissatisfaction: A survey of relatives of intensive care patients who died." *Crit. Care Med.* 26, 7: 1187–93.

Marion, R. 1989. *The Intern Blues*. New York: Ballantine Books.

Max, M.B., and R.K. Portenoy. 1998. "Pain research: Designing clinical trials in palliative care." In Doyle, Hanks, and MacDonald, eds., *Oxford Textbook of Palliative Medicine*.

McCue, J. 1995. "The naturalness of dying." *JAMA* 13, 273: 1034–43.

McCormick, W., T. Inui, R. Deyo, et al. 1991. "Long term care preferences of hospitalized patients with AIDS." *J. Gen. Intern. Med.* 6: 524–8.

McFarlane, T.J., ed. 2003. *Einstein and Buddha: The Parallel Sayings*. Berkeley, CA: Ulysses Press.

McGovern, G., 1996. *Terry*. New York: Villard Books.

McKay, M., and Fanning, P. 1987. *Self Esteem*. Oakland, CA: New Harbinger Publications.

McNees, P. ed. 1996. *Dying: A Book of Comfort*. New York: Warner Books.

McWhinney, I.R., and M.A. Stewart. 1994. "Home care for dying patients. Family physicians' experience with a palliative care support team." *Can Fam. Physician* 40: 240–6.

Merriman, M.P. 1999. "Documenting the impact of hospice." *The Hospice Journal* 14, 314: 177–92.

Miller, W.R., et al. 1995. *Motivational Enhancement Therapy Manual*. Project MATCH Monograph Series. Volume 2. US Department of Health and Human Services, Public Health Services, National Institute of Health, 67–86.

Mitchell, G. 1998. "Assessment of GP management of symptoms of dying patients in an Australian community hospice by chart audit." *Fam. Pract.* 15: 420–5.

Morin, C.M., and N.H. Azin. 1987. "Stimulus control and imagery training in treating sleep maintenance insomnia." *J. Consult. Clin. Psychol.* 55, 2: 260–2.

Morin, C.M., J.P. Culbert, and S.M. Schwartz. 1994. "Non-pharmacological interventions for insomnia: A meta-analysis of treatment efficacy." *Am. J. Psychiatry* 151, 8: 1172–80.

Morrison, M.F. 1998. "Obstacles to doctor-patient communication at the end of life." In M.D. Steinberg and S.J. Youngner, eds. *End-of-life Decisions: A Psychosocial Perspective*. Washington, DC: American Psychiatric Press.

Morrison, R.S., E.W. Morrisson, and D.F. Glickman. 1994. "Physician reluctance to discuss advance directives: An empiric investigation of potential barriers." *Arch. Intern. Med.* 154: 2311–18.

Morrison, R.S., L.H. Zayas, M. Mulvihill, et al. 1998. "Barriers to completion of health care proxies." *Arch. Intern. Med.* 158: 2493–7.

Mount, B.M., and J.F. Scott. 1983. "Whither hospice evaluation?" *J. Chronic Dis.* 36: 731–6.

Murphy, S., J. Palmer, S. Azen, et al. 1996. "Ethnicity and advance directives." *J. Law Med. Ethics*, 24: 108–17.

Murtagh, D.R., and K.M. Greenwood. 1995. "Identifying effective psychological treatments for insomnia: A meta-analysis." *J. Consult. Coin. Psychol.* 63, 1: 79–89.

Mynors-Wallis, L.M., D.H. Gath, A.R. Lloyd-Thomas, et al. 1995. "Randomized controlled trial comparing problem solving treatment with amitryptine and placebo for major depression in primary care." *BMJ* 310: 441–5.

National Heart, Lung, and Blood Institute. 1995. "What is insomnia?" NIH Publication No. 95-3801.

National Hospice Organization. 1996. "Hospice awareness campaign 'Handle with Care' needs your participation." *NHO Newsline* 7, 15: 1.

National Institute on Alcohol Abuse and Alcoholism (NIAAA). 1992. *Alcohol Alert: Moderate Drinking.* Bethesda, MD, National Institute on Alcohol Abuse and Alcoholism, No.16 PH 315.

– 1995. *The Physicians' Guide to Helping Patients with Alcohol Problems.* Bethesda, MD: National Institute on Alcohol Abuse and Alcoholism, NIH Publication No. 95-3769.

– 2003. *FAQs on alcohol abuse and alcoholism.* www.niaaa.nih.gov/faq/q-a.htm.

Nimocks, M.J.A., L. Webb, and J.R. Connell. 1987. "Communication and the terminally ill: A theoretical model." *Death Stud.* 11: 323–44.

North, C.S., and J.M. Ryan. 1997. "Psychiatric illness in female physicians." *Postgrad. Med.* 101, 5: 233–42.

Northwest Territories Bureau of Statistics. 1996. "1996 NWT Alcohol and Drug Survey: Rates of use for alcohol, other drugs and tobacco." www.stats.gov.nt.ca/Statinfo/health/alcdrug/report.html

Nuland, S. 1995. *How We Die: Reflections on Life's Final Chapter.* New York: Vintage Books.

Odoi, L.F., and V.R. Cassidy. 1998. "The message of SUPPORT: Change is long overdue." *J. Prof. Nurs.* 14, 3: 165–74.

Parkes, C.M. 1998. "Bereavement." In Doyle, Hanks, and MacDonald, eds., *Oxford Textbook of Palliative Medicine.*

Parkes, C.M., and R.S. Weiss. 1983. *Recovery from Bereavement.* New York: Basic Books.

Peabody, B. 1987. *The Screaming Room: A Mother's Journal of Her Son's Struggle With AIDS.* New York: Avon.

Peck, M.S. 1986. *The Road Less Traveled.* New York: Simon and Schuster.

Pennebaker, J. 1990. *Opening Up: The Healing Power of Confiding in Others.* New York: Avon.

Penson, R.J., K.M. Green, et al. 2002. "When does the responsibility of our care end: Bereavement." *The Oncologist* 7: 251–8.

Pfeifer, M.P., J.E. Sidorov, A.C. Smith, et al. 1994. "The discussion of end-of-life medical care by primary care patients and physicians: A multi centre study using qualitative interviews." *J. Gen. Intern. Med.* 9: 82–8.

Placek, J.T., and T.L. Eberhardt. 1996. "Breaking bad news." *JAMA* 276, 6: 496–502.

Portenoy, R.K., H.T. Thaler, A.B. Kornblith, et al. 1994. "Symptom prevalence, characteristics and distress in a cancer population." *Qual. Life Res.* 3: 183–9.

Potter-Effron, R., and P. Potter-Effron. 1989. *Letting Go of Shame: Understanding How Shame Affects Your Life.* Center City, MN: Hazelden.

Pradko, J.F., and A.J. Rush. 1999. "Depression: Beyond stereotype and stigma: A CME Monograph." Little Faus, NJ: Projects in Knowledge, 1999.

Prather, H. 1970. *Notes to Myself.* Lafayette, CA: Real People Press.

Prescott, B.J. "The Terminally Ill Child." In A.D. Lester., ed. *When Children Suffer: a Sourcebook for Ministry with Children in Crisis.* Louisville, KY: Westminster John Knox Press.

Prigerson, H.G., and S.C. Jacobs. 2001. "Caring for bereaved patients: 'All the doctors just suddenly go.'" *JAMA* 286: 1369–76.

Pritchard, R.S., E.S. Fisher, J.M. Teno, et al. 1998. *J. Am. Geriatr. Soc.* 46: 1242–50.

Progoff, I. 1975. *At a Journal Workshop.* New York: Tarcher/Putnam.

Quill, T.E. 2000. "Initiating end-of-life discussions with seriously ill patients." *JAMA* 284,19: 2502–7

Quill, T.E., R. Dresser, and D.W. Brock. 1997. "The rule of double effect – a critique of its role in end-of-life decision making." *N. Engl. J. Med.* 337, 24: 1768–71.

Rabow, M.W., G.E. Hardie, J.M. Fair, et al. 2000. "End-of-life care content in 50 textbooks from multiple specialties." *JAMA* 283, 6: 771–8.

Raffin, T.A. 1995. "Withdrawing life support: How is the decision made?" *JAMA* 273: 738–9.

Remen, R.N. 1997. "Caring spirit." *Living Fit.* August: 120

Reuben, D.B. 1989. "Depressive symptoms in medical house officers." *Arch. Intern. Med.* 145: 286–8.

Richards, M.C. 1989. *Centering in Pottery, Poetry and the Person.* Middletown, CT: Wesleyan University Press.

Rinpoche, S. 1992. *The Tibetan Book of Living and Dying.* New York: Harper Collins.

Roberts, W.O., S. DeMann, and R.D. Durand. "Insomnia: Treatment options for the 21st century." *Postgrad. Med. A Special Report* (no vol.): 1–55

Roth, T. 2000. "Overview of insomnia for the primary care physician." In Roberts, DeMann, and Durand, eds., "Insomnia: Treatment options for the 21st century," 5-13.

Rousseau, P. 2001. "Caring for the dying: Why is it so hard for physicians?" *West J. Med.* 175: 284–5.

Rutkowski, A. 2002. "Death notification in the emergency department." *Ann. Emerg. Med.* 40: 521–3.

Sachs, G.A. 1998. "Opportunities for promoting palliative medicine in cancer research." *Cancer Investigation* 16, 7: 503–8.

Samkoft, J., S. Hockenberry, L.L. Simon, et al. 1995. "Mortality of young physicians in the US, 1980–1988." *Acad. Med.* 70: 242–4.

Schaefer, C., C.P. Quesenberry, Jr., S. Wi. 1995. "Mortality following conjugal bereavement and the effects of a shared environment." *Am. J. Epidemiol.* 141: 1142–52.

Scheel, B.Y., and J. Lynn. 1988. "Care of dying patients." *Clinics in Geriatrics* 4, 3: 639–55.

Scheidman, E.S. 1980. *Voices of Man.* New York: Harper and Row.

Schneiderman, L.J. 1997. "The family physician and end-of-life care." *J. Fam. Pract.* 45, 3: 259–62.

Schneiderman, L.J., R.M. Kaplan, R.A. Pearlman, et al. 1993. "Do physicians own preferences for life-sustaining treatment influence their perceptions of patients' preferences?" *J. Clin. Ethics* 4: 28–33.

Schonwetter, R.S., ed. 1999. "Hospice and palliative medicine: Philosophy, history, and standards of care." In *Hospice and Palliative Medicine: Core Curriculum and Review Syllabus.* Dubuque, Iowa: Kendall/Hunt.

Seckler, A.B., D.E. Meier, M. Mulvihill, et al. 1991. "Substituted judgment: How accurate are proxy predictions?" *Ann. Intern. Med.* 115: 92–8.

Shields, C.F. 1998. "Giving patients bad news." *Primary Care* 25, 2: 381–90.

Shuster, J.L., W. Breitbart, and H. Chochinov. 1999. "Psychiatric aspects of excellent end-of-life care." *Psychosomatics* 40, 1: 1–3.

Siegel, B.S. 1986. *Love, Medicine, and Miracles.* New York: Harper and Row.

Siegler, E.L., and B.W. Levin. 2000. "Physician-older patient communication at the end of life." *Clin. Geriatr. Med.* 16: 175–204.

Simon, R.D. 2000. "Tailoring the treatment of insomnia to the individual patient." In Roberts, DeMann, and Durand, eds. "Insomnia: Treatment options for the 21st century," 41–54.

Simonton, O.C., S. Matthews-Simonton, and J. Creighton. 1978. *Getting Well Again.* Toronto: Bantam Books.

Singer, P.A., D.K. Martin, and M. Kelner. 1999. "Quality end-of-life care. Patients' perspectives." *JAMA* 281, 2: 163–8.

Slevin, M.L., L. Stubbs, H.J. Plant, et al. 1990. "Attitudes to chemotherapy: comparing views of patients with cancer with those of doctors, nurses, and general public." *BMJ* 300, 6737: 1458–60.

Smith, T.J., and K. Swisher. 1998. "Telling the truth about terminal cancer." *JAMA* 279, 21: 1746–8.

Steinmetz, D., et al. 1992. "The family physician's role in caring for the dying patient and family: A comprehensive, theoretical model." *Fam. Pract.* 9: 433–6.

Stevens M. 1998. "The psychological adaptation of the dying child." In Doyle, Hanks, MacDonald, eds., *The Oxford Textbook of Palliative Medicine.*

Stolick, M. 2002. "Overcoming the tendency to lie to dying patients." *Am. J. Hosp. Palliat. Care* 19: 29–34.

Storey, P., and C.F. Knight. 1996. *UNIPAC Four: Management of Selected Nonpain Symptoms in the Terminally Ill.* Dubuque, Iowa: Kendall/Hunt Publishing.

– 1998. *UNIPAC One: The Hospice/Palliative Medicine Approach in End-of-Life Care.* Dubuque, Iowa: Kendall/Hunt Publishing.

– 2003. *UNIPAC Three: Assessment and Treatment of Pain in the Terminally Ill.* (2nd ed.) Larchmont, NY: Mary Ann Liebert, Publishers.

Substance Abuse and Mental Health Services Administration (SAMHSA). 2003. "The National Survey on Drug Use and Health: The NSDUH Report. Quantity and frequency of alcohol use." www.oas.samhsa.gov/2k3/AlcQF/AlcQF.htm

Sulmasy, D.P., K. Haller, and P. Terry. 1994. "More talk, less paper: Predicting the accuracy of substituted judgments." *Am. J. Med.* 96: 432–8.

Sundquist, J., and S. Johansson. 1999. "Impaired health status and mental health, lower vitality, and social functioning in women general practitioners in Sweden." *Scand. J. Prim. Health Care.* 17: 81–6

SUPPORT Principal Investigators. 1995. "A controlled trial to improve care for seriously ill hospitalized patients: The study to understand prognoses and preferences for outcomes and risks of treatment (SUPPORT)." *JAMA* 274: 1591–8.

Swanson, J., and A. Cooper. 1994. *The Complete Relapse Prevention Skills Program.* Part I. Center City, MN: Hazelden.

Swanson, J., and A. Cooper. 1995. *The Complete Relapse Prevention Skills Program.* Part II. Center City, MN: Hazelden.

Task Force on DSM-IV. 2000. *Diagnostic and Statistical Manual of Mental Disorders.* DSM-IV-TR *(Text Revision).* Washington, DC: American Psychiatric Association.

Tempero, M.A. 1997. "Walking a difficult path is easier with a friend. Thoughts from a practicing oncologist." *Ann. N.Y. Acad. Sci.* 809: 237–42.

Teno, J., J. Fleishman, D.W. Borck, et al. 1990. "The use of formal prior directives among patients with HIV-related diseases." *J. Gen. Intern. Med.* 5: 490–4.

Tierney, R.M., and S.M. Horton. 1998. "Relationships between symptom relief, quality of life, and satisfaction with hospice care." *Palliat. Med.* 12: 333–44.

Tinseley, E.S., et al. 1994. *Surgeons, nurses, and bereaved families' attitudes toward dying in the burn centre.* Professor R.F. Edlich, Department of Plastic Surgery, Box 332, Charlottesville, VA. 22908.

Torrecilas, L. 1997. "Communication of the cancer diagnosis to Mexican patients." *Ann. N.Y. Acad. Sci.* 809: 188–96.

Towsend, J., A.D. Frank, and D. Fermont, et al. 1990. "Terminal cancer care and patients' preference for place of death: A prospective study." *BMJ* 301: 415–17.

Trimm, F. 1995. "Divorce and death: Helping children cope with family loss." *Comprehensive Therapy* 21, 3: 135–8.

Twycross, R., and I. Lichter. 1988. "Plenary Session: How whole is our Care?" Address to the Seventh International Congress on Care of the Terminally Ill, Montreal. Quoted in Adams, D.W., and E.J. Deveau, eds. 1995. *The Innocence of Childhood: Helping children and Adolescents Cope with Life-Threatening Illness and Dying.* Amityville, NY: Baywood Publishing.

Twycross, R., and I. Lichter. 1998 "The terminal phase." In Doyle, Hanks, MacDonald, eds. *Oxford Textbook of Palliative Medicine.*

US Department of Health and Human Services Public Health Service. 1995. NIH Publication No. 95-3801. Bethseda, MD: National Institutes of Health: National Heart, Lung, and Blood Institute.

Vachon, M.L.S. 1995. "Staff stress in hospice/palliative care: A review." *Palliat. Med.* 9: 91–122.

– 1998. "The stress of professional caregivers." In Doyle, Hanks, MacDonald, eds., *Oxford Textbook of Palliative Medicine.*

Varner, K.S., ed. 1998. *Curriculum Directory.* Washington, DC: Association of American Medical Colleges.

Verghese, A. 1995. *My Own Country.* New York: Random House.

Voltz, R., and G.D. Borasio. 1997. "Palliative therapy in the terminal stage of neurological disease." *J. Neurol.* 244. Supplement 4: S2–S10.

von Gunten, C.F., J.H. Von Foenn, K.J. Neely, et al. 1995. "Hospice and palliative care: Attitudes and practices of the physician faculty of an academic hospital." *Am. J. Hosp. Palliat. Care* 12: 38–2.

von Gunten, C.F., F.D. Ferris, and L.L. Emanuel. 2000. "Ensuring competency in end-of-life care." *JAMA* 284, 23: 3051–7.

Walsh, J.K., R.M. Benca, M. Bonnet, et al. 1998. "Insomnia: Assessment and management in primary care." Bethesda, MD: National Heart, Lung, and Blood Institute. NIH Publication no. 98-4088.

Walters, D., and J. Tupin. 1991. "Family grief in the emergency department." *Emerg. Med. Clin. North Am.* 9, 1: 189–207.

Wear, D. 2002. "'Face to face with it': Medical students' narratives about their end-of-life education." *Acad. Med.* 77: 271–7.

Weinman Lear, M. 1980. *Heartsounds.* New York: Simon and Schuster.

Wenrich, M.D., J.R. Curtis, and S.E. Shannon. 2001. "Communicating with dying patients within the spectrum of medical care from terminal diagnosis to death." *Arch. Intern. Med.* 161: 868–74.

Werch, C.E., D.R. Gorman, and P.J. Marty. 1987. "Relationship between alcohol consumption and alcohol problems in young adults." *J. Drug Ed.* 17, 3: 261–76.

White, R., and M. Cunningham. 1992. *My Own Story*. New York: Penguin Books.

Whitten, J.R. 1998. "Ten commandments for the care of terminally ill patients." *Am. Fam. Physician* 57, 5: 935–40.

Worden, J.W. 1996. *Children and Grief: When a Parent Dies*. New York: Guilford.

– 2002. *Grief Counseling and Grief Therapy*. New York: Springer Publishing.

Yates, P. 1993. "Towards a re-conceptualization of hope for patients with a diagnosis of cancer." *J. Adv. Nurs.* 18: 701–6.

Zeitlin, S. 2001. "Grief and bereavement." *Primary Care: Clinics in Office Practise* 28: 415–25.

Index